Praise for

M000288974

~~Lie~~

"Nick Delgado is a prolific science writer and nutrition expert in the science of human performance sports. He contributes his expertise in this new book, *Blood Doesn't Lie.* He is a pioneering member of the preventive and alternative medicine movement with special expertise in nutritional health and elite sports performance. What he says works not simply because he's done a respectable job of researching the facts but because he applies this technology to himself and to his clients, who are themselves elite athletes. Nick brings a wealth of real-world expertise to the topic and his opinions are worthy of attention."

Dr. Ron Klatz MD DO is a physician, medical scientist, inventor, President and founder of the American Academy of Anti-Aging Medicine-A4M (nonprofit), and Founder of the National Academy of Sports Medicine – NASM. He has over 30 years in the fitness industry with Dr. Bob Goldman. He is executive medical editor of the *Encyclopedia of Clinical Anti-Aging Medicine & Regenerative Biomedical Technologies* and author of *Infection Protection.* http://Worldhealth.net

"In *Blood Doesn't Lie*, you'll learn about promising, all-natural therapies for preventing and promoting recovery from even the most severe infections. One example out of many in the book is how to strengthen the lymphatic system and how to dramatically increase the production of white blood cells called B-lymphocytes, which produce antibodies that offer protection from multiple types of illnesses. The information in this book is highly important."

Anil Bajnath, MD, MBA, IFMCP, ABAARM, MIFHI, Adjunct Assistant Professor, Department of Clinical Research and Leadership, George Washington University School of Medicine and Health Sciences, Founder & CEO, The Institute for Human Optimization https://ifho.org

"The cliché' that 'health is the greatest wealth' is tautologically true. To be optimally healthy, you need to have a *sustainably perfected immune system.* My longtime friend and trusted colleague, Nick Delgado, practices what he preaches, has healed himself from death's door and done so for many others. Now he has a perfected immune system builder to keep you healthy all the days of your life."

Mark Victor Hansen, Co-creator of *Chicken Soup for the Soul*, and the *One Minute Millionaire*, and *ASK!* series.

"How timely to re-emphasize with scientific forcefulness the critical role of the mind/body connection. As a man thinketh, so is he (Proverbs 23:7) and his immune system will be, hence the new field of psychoneuroimmunology. Nick Delgado, a diet and fitness expert, truly walks the walk and gives us his nutritional, fitness, and other healthy aging secrets for enhancing our own immune system and preventing ANY disease. Succinct, well-written and documented and could be life-saving!"

Joseph C. Maroon, MD, Clinical Professor of neurological surgery, nutritional and health expert, Ironman triathlete. Dr Maroon has been the team neurosurgeon for the Pittsburgh Steelers since 1981 and is Medical Director of World Wrestling Entertainment (WWE).

"*Blood Doesn't Lie* gets to the core of how to build a strong immune system with the hormones you need to optimize and safeguard yourself from infectious diseases and the roles stem cells, peptides, cortisol, and mitochondria play in disease prevention and reversal. It's highly informative and easy to follow!"

Dr. Cathleen Gerenger, DC in Tampa, Florida. She graduated from Life University/Life Chiropractic College/West Campus in 1998 and specializes in acupuncture, and sports medicine at RaJeunir Medical Center.

"Do you want to have a stronger immune system? Teach everyone the lifestyle medicine hacks provided in this book! With a wealth of experience in the preventative medicine industry, researching, educating doctors, and coaching elite clients towards optimal health, Nick's level of expertise is unsurpassed. What makes *Blood Doesn't Lie* so effective and revolutionary is the fact that it details diet and lifestyle protocols to not only bolster immune defenses but also optimize all the other systems and organs in the body that play supportive roles in immunity. *Blood Doesn't Lie* is your best defense against infectious diseases, and your greatest ally in the pursuit of a long, healthy life."

Michael Grossman MD is a graduate of New York University School of Medicine and a Diplomat of the American Board of Family Practice. He was an Assistant Clinical Professor at the University of California at Irvine School of Medicine.
OCwellness.com

"The immune system does not function as an island; it is reliant on many other systems and organs in the body. Preventative medicine pioneer Nick Delgado understands this. He takes a holistic, multi-pronged, evidence-based approach to immune health and shares it in this book for the world to benefit! This is arguably the most thorough and advanced guide to optimal immunity ever written and with pandemics on the rise, *Blood Doesn't Lie* couldn't have come at a better time!"

Maryanne A. Hannaney, MD, FACOG, FAARFM. She is affiliated with Hoag Memorial Hospital Presbyterian

"This book talks about what modern medicine isn't discussing--that our immune systems and natural body processes, when healthy, are defense systems. The information in this book will help you to understand how your immune system works, the truth about viruses, and how to set yourself up to stay healthy and any to come. I have been telling my clients for years that food is medicine and now I can refer them to this book for the science behind that claim."

Leah Grant, Master Certified Coach, is a Training Director and a leading coach for high-level financial advisers and advisory teams in the US. She is also a Certified Emotional Intelligence Practitioner, and a Certified NLP Practitioner.

"An optimally functioning immune system is your absolute best defense against infectious diseases and this much-needed book reveals the exact steps you need to take to achieve it. Nick Delgado is a pioneering member of the preventive medicine movement, and *Blood Doesn't Lie* is a compilation of all the knowledge he's gained in over 40 years of research and clinical practice. Nick's protocols are both cutting edge and comprehensive, and you will learn everything from nutritional and herbal therapy, to stem cell and mitochondrial optimization, to the importance of detoxification and adrenal support. *Blood Doesn't Lie* is not only your best defense against infectious diseases but also your greatest ally in the pursuit of a long, healthy life!"

Sangeeta Pati, MD is a holistic medicine specialist in Orlando, Florida. SAJUNE Institute for Restorative and Regenerative Medicine in Orlando, Florida specializes in Hormone Optimization, Nutrition and Weight Management.

Blood Doesn't Lie

Nick Delgado, PhD, ABAAHP, CHT

Blood Doesn't Lie
By Nick Delgado PhD, ABAAHP, CHT

Copyright 2020 Nick Delgado, PhD ABAAHP CHT
Published by
Health Wellness Studios, Inc.

ISBN: 978-0-9962196-2-4
Printed in the United States of America

All Rights Reserved

All rights reserved. Except as permitted by applicable copyright laws, no part of this book may be reproduced, duplicated, sold or distributed in any form or by any means, either mechanical, by photocopy, electronic, or by computer, or stored in a database or retrieval system, without the express written permission of the publisher/authors, except for brief quotations by reviewers.

This book is not intended to provide medical advice or to take the place of medical advice and treatment from your personal physician. Readers are advised to consult their own doctors or other qualified health professionals regarding the treatment of their medical problems. Neither the publisher nor the authors take any responsibility for any possible consequences from any treatment, action or application of medicine, supplement, herb, or preparation to any person reading or following information in this book. If readers take prescription medications, again, they should consult with their physicians and not take themselves off medicines to start supplementations or a nutrition program without proper supervision of a physician.

We do not directly endorse any company or product. We align with strategic partnerships to promote wellness, prevention, and education, the triad necessary for lifestyle medicine. There may be areas of conflicting or promising data between modern medicine and holistic therapies, proof that more studies are needed. Final conclusions may be challenging given the scarcity of information, limitations in research design, and flawed data. We present our interpretation of just some of the existing data.

Table of Contents

About the Author

I want to share with you why I wrote this book. I previously suffered with a weakened immune system which led me to search the world for the answers that you are about to learn. In writing this book I have literally drawn upon over 1,000 interviews that I have collected from over 26,000 leading researchers and scientists to help design the best approach to immune rejuvenation. I wrote abstracts and blogs with my team of experts and presented my findings to doctors and scientists all over the world at medical and nutritional conferences.

I was not always healthy. My first 23 years of life were filled with health struggles. At the age of 12, I was not only extremely overweight, I also suffered with irritable bowel syndrome. I went to a doctor who didn't believe I was having diarrhea every day. I left dismayed however I went to the medical library and found a nutrition textbook that helped me understand more about digestive health. I discovered Latins, Asians, and Blacks react more severely than other races to yogurt, cheese, whole and even nonfat cows milk. I realized these foods were making my condition worse and within a few days of eliminating all dairy from my diet, the loose bowels were solved.

My health struggles didn't end there though. From the age of 16 to 22, I struggled with hypertension, skin conditions, hormonal imbalances including estrogen dominance, excessive overeating, and a body fat level of over 25%. Most of these problems were solved with a plant-based, oil-free, sugar-free diet, which I implemented after meeting and studying with Nathan Pritikin. I also studied with the German doctor, Ron Duvendack, MD. He taught me the importance of monitoring the immune system, and how to do so with blood microscopy, and white blood cell, liver, kidney, and lipid metabolism analysis.

I learned how whole plant-based foods can alter inflammatory antigens and how the correct combination of herbs and foods helps to build a healthier immune system. I also learned the importance of using delayed food testing in order to identify potentially intolerant foods. The body may view common foods you consume as foreign proteins which can make even the healthiest of foods damaging to your body, and this is particularly common in people with autoimmune diseases.

Adrenal fatigue was another huge piece of the puzzle of immune depression that I discovered. If you get sick often, experience cravings or addictions, or have ongoing fatigue ask yourself the following:

Do you feel tired even after a good night's sleep?

Do you find it difficult to recover after exercise, especially after participating in extreme sports?

Do you have constant colds, flu, and bronchitis that have lasted months which prevents you from being able to exercise consistently?

If you answered yes to any of the above, adrenal fatigue is likely to blame.

For over 40 years I have been gathering more pieces of the puzzle through research, clinical practice, anti-aging conferences, and lifestyle medicine events. I also gained essential insights during my studies alongside some of the world's leading endocrinology interventionists including Thierry Hertoghe, MD, UC San Diego Professor Ron Rothenberg, Jonathan Wright, MD, Edwin Lee, MD, and several others. They have all published several textbooks on hormone management and longevity. I applied our collective findings to our clients and used lifestyle medicine (herbs, sleep hygiene, stem cells, mitochondrial support, etc) to improve hormone balance, overcome estrogen dominance and adrenal fatigue, and rejuvenate the immune system.

This was amazing, yet I discovered the ability to guide people on their journey toward optimal health is best accomplished with the science of epigenetics. I continued to mentor students and doctors while I became a high-level life mastery coach for Tony Robbins Mastery University. My work with Tad James, Bruce Lipton, Ph.D., and Mark Victor Hansen, Author of Chicken Soup for the Soul, the Ask series, and the number one trainer in TimeLine Therapy, helped me to realize that when we include the power of the subconscious mind, we can help millions of people transform their lives.

The proper integration of each of these therapies allowed for a personalized plan that was reproducible. The turnaround in my health even though I am past the age of 65 has included my participation in extreme nonstop weight-lifting sports which I love. My immune system according to most of my doctor friends is extraordinary. Optimizing my clients' health, many of whom are famous doctors, fitness stars, and executives who are past the age of 60, 70, 80, or even 90 has been an incredible journey!

To help make optimal health accessible to the masses, I started offering affordable online courses, and podcasts that are aired on Spotify, iTunes, and YouTube, which is approaching 2 million views. Our coaching program is now personalized for each person based on their goals. Hormonal imbalances, acne, estrogen dominance, chronic fatigue, inflammatory conditions, cancer, respiratory distress, and those with depressed immune systems can and have been helped. This book *Blood Doesn't Lie* is the most exciting guide to take beginners and even advanced enthusiasts of health to the next level with the most effective and advanced, yet surprisingly simple lifestyle medicine solutions.

Nick Delgado, ABAAHP (American Board of Anti-Aging Health Practitioners) is a forerunner of today's

Lifestyle Medicine movement with over 43 years of clinical experience.

Nick is the author of Grow Young and Slim eBook, and Simply Healthy Vegan Cookbook; and the coauthor of Acne Be Gone for Good, along with Sonia Badreshia Bansal, MD, dermatologist. He is also the author of Mastering Love, Sex, and Intimacy, which is endorsed by John Gray, author of Men are from Mars - Women are from Venus.

Nick has always strived to present practical solutions to challenging health problems. His YouTube channel is http://Youtube.com/DelgadoVideo.

His best shows connect to http://NickDelgado.com

His clients achieve outstanding results, and he is known as the guide who is not afraid to share the truth. Ray Wilson, the founder of Family Fitness, says Nick is the person who is best suited to "lead and mentor those who want to be heroes in their lifetime."

Nick's mission is to lead the health care system and media to help those struggling with chronic diseases of aging or deficiencies which are preventable or even reversible. Enjoy this book *Blood Doesn't Lie* and share it with all of those you care about!

With *Blood Doesn't Lie* I can now help people strengthen their immune systems within days. The methods in this book support the body's production of over 6 million white blood cells per minute, which form antibodies with nearly one billion combinations to protect us from microbes, fungi, viruses, bacteria, and toxins!

My Story

Why Health and Nutrition is so important to me

Though I was a lifelong athlete and was following what was conventionally thought of as a Healthy American Diet. At 23 I suffered a transient ischemic attack(a "mild" stroke). From that day forward I chose to dedicate my life to finding out what was actually healthy and living my life in a way that put what I learned into practice. In the next several months the weight that I struggled with for years fell off, losing more than 55 pounds in five months which along with my blood pressure medication I have kept off ever since.

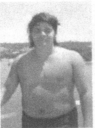

Nick Delgado, 210 lbs at a height of 5'8

As you can see, the results speak for themselves. Below and to the right are pictures of me following My own Coaching Program and hyper nutrient dense eating and supplementation protocols

Nick Delgado, 155 lbs lean and fit after committing his life to health and wellness

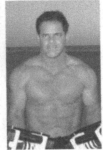

Nick Delgado, 180 lbs age 52, on the Delgado Protocol

Dr Nick & Anil MD, 43 years of Microscopy & 20 years studying and working to enhance the immune system and circulation.

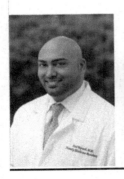

Chicken

Under

Microscope

NICK**DELGADO**

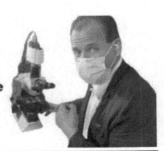

Introduction

The most effective way to protect ourselves from infectious diseases or chronic degenerative diseases is to understand the concepts of proactive intervention, preventative medicine, and lifestyle support. We have a powerful, intelligent immune system that is designed to always withstand toxic microbial inundation.

Medicine has evolved dramatically even compared with 20 years ago, but every new disease requires a new response. Infectious diseases can spread quickly to many patients, warns Tasuku Honjo, a Japanese physician-scientist, immunologist, and Nobel prize winner.

Although normal bodily defense systems play a significant preventative role, they are not the only things needed to stop a virulent disease. We also have several white blood cells including the B-cells, T-cells, and natural killer cells, which can mount an incredible defense against any foreign invader. All these defenses are components of the immune system. The immune system is more extensive than the entire circulatory system. It includes our lymph glands and the antibodies that are transported not only by our blood circulation but also by the immune system's own lymph fluid transport system.

Exposure to pathogens plays an important role in the building of a robust immune system. It allows our immune systems to build antibodies and other defenses to protect us. This is not to say we should go out of our way to try to get sick; actually quite the opposite: support your immune system with guidelines in this book and then let it do its job by living life to the fullest.

Imagine you had an American football team that planned to play against the best defensive team in the league, but they showed up with no offensive linemen and without any protection for their quarterback and running backs. Even with the best quarterback in the league and fastest running backs, they could not last more than a few plays before the big defensive lineman (bacteria) and linebackers (viruses) swarmed all over the quarterback or running backs (brain, lungs, and immune system). Before long, the team would be weakened, fatigued, battered, and bruised to the point where they would lose the battle.

The sick and elderly, those with chronic illnesses, and those with chronic fatigue can be likened to this football team; they do not have the immune defenses to fight pathogens. These high-risk people will benefit the most from the protocols laid out in this book, which include nutrification, detoxification, hormonal and herbal support, and power of the mind. This book wasn't written just for older people however, it was written for everyone.

We in America rank 36th in the world in life expectancy and we have more sick days than many other countries. This reflects our toxic diets and sedentary, high-stress lifestyles, and it's time we took responsibility for our health and made better choices. My clients, my children, my 85-year-old mother, my staff, and I have all implemented these protocols for a superhero immune system with great success and now you can too! As the saying goes you either invest in your health now, or you will pay later. Spending a few extra dollars on healthy food and nutraceuticals could mean saving hundreds of thousands of dollars down the road on doctors, hospitals, and insurance premiums.

In this book, you will learn safe, all-natural ways to optimize your immune system to reduce your risk of contracting pathogens and minimize symptoms if you do. You will also learn why people around the world are seeking more natural solutions and breakthrough treatment methods to support rapid healing. With the multifaceted approach outlined in this book, we can dramatically reduce the recovery time from infections; cut missed workdays in half and win the battle against infectious diseases!

Section 1:

The Immune System

–

Your Best Defense

Chapter 1:

The Intricate and Powerful Immune System

The Immune System Superheroes

"What do you think you have an immune system for - it's for killing germs!" George Carlin - YouTube: Germs, Immune System

You are not helpless against disease. Whether or not you become infected and critically ill is not a matter of fate: established research shows that immune dysfunction plays a central role in this process. Imbalances and dysfunctions of the immune system place you at a much greater risk for severe infections. The best way to protect yourself from infectious diseases is to maintain a robust immune system. When the immune system is functioning optimally, most pathogens are no longer a threat because the immune system will destroy them before they can hijack the cells.

White Blood Cells - Your Frontline Defense

One of the vital defense mechanisms of the immune system is the white blood cells (also known as leukocytes). The white blood cells and antibodies can adjust to over one million different "mutant germs." There are five major types of white blood cells: neutrophils, eosinophils, basophils, monocytes, and lymphocytes.

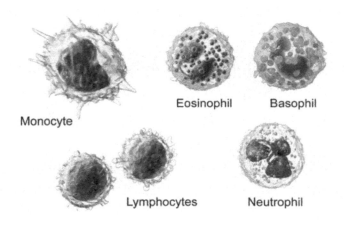

Neutrophils and monocytes engulf foreign pathogens and destroy them. Lymphocytes, which include the T cells and B cells, are a type of white blood cell that identifies pathogens so that the immune system can generate specific antibodies against that particular pathogen, and they are our first line of defense against new viral invaders. Natural killer cells (another type of lymphocyte) detect diseases and kill virally infected cells

White Blood Cell Quantity and Efficiency

Examples of Bad White Blood Cell Quantity Under the Microscope
Excessive number of white blood cells triggered by viral exposure or food incompatibility can start destroying healthy tissue too

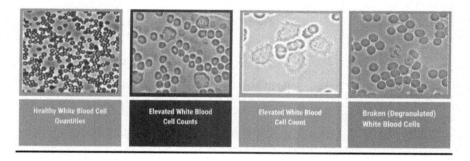

| Healthy White Blood Cell Quantities | Elevated White Blood Cell Counts | Elevated White Blood Cell Count | Broken (Degranulated) White Blood Cells |

White blood cell quantity is an indicator of the health of your immune system. If your immune system is overactive, it can lead to an elevated white blood cell count, and cells that have self-destructed to save you from a threat that wasn't real. If it is underactive, there will be fewer white blood cells in your blood.

Examples of High and Low White Blood Cell Efficiency Under the Microscope
We develop strong immune systems with proper support based on millions of years of our bodies learning to combat invading toxins, bacteria and viruses. The proper hormone levels, physical activity, outdoor daylight, sleep and herbs all play a role in our health

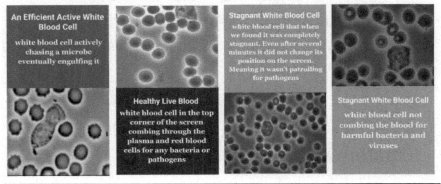

Antibodies

Antibodies are proteins produced from the B lymphocytes which recognize and bind to invading pathogens, thus neutralizing them. Each of us has five different isotypes of antibodies (IgM, IgD, IgG, IgA and IgE). IgG is the most abundant antibody isotype in the blood plasma accounting for 70-75% of human immunoglobulins (antibodies).

It is estimated that humans can generate about 10 billion different antibodies, each capable of binding to a distinct epitope of an antigen. At this point the pathogen is no longer capable of infecting the host -- you! Over time the antibodies will gradually disappear, while the memory B cells will remain dormant in your body for many years, yet ready to activate if a similar invader appears. This is what we mean when we say the body has built an immunity to a particular pathogen and this is how we gain immunity.

B cells - produce one type of antibody for 1 foreign molecule, with a **billion** different types of B cells to handle a variety of potential pathogens on the planet! When attacked by a virus, within minutes, the B cells divide into swarms of clones to produce **millions of antibodies** to defend against the toxic virus.

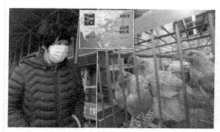
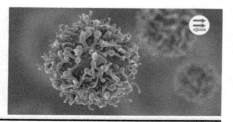

Compromised Immunity and Risk

Unfortunately for the elderly, vital immune cells naturally decline with age - this is why the elderly and sick are at a much higher risk for severe illness. Also, because the modern diet and lifestyle are so toxic, a large proportion of non-elderly people have compromised immune systems that are either underactive or overactive.[1] When the immune system is underactive, it often leads to a shortage of one or more of the immune system- supporting white blood cells, which grossly inhibits the body's ability to defend

---

[1]

https://www.betterhealth.vic.gov.au/health/ConditionsAndTreatments/immune-system?viewAsPdf=true itself from infectious diseases. This places a person at a much higher risk for contracting a disease and will lead to more severe symptoms and slower recovery if they do. Now for some good news - data from over 43 years of blood microscopy shows that we can boost our immune system ten-fold in as little as three days using strategies which are outlined in the next critical chapters of this book.

Chapter 2:

Eating Animals Causes Disease

Animals are a major cause of global infectious disease. We need to stop eating animals or dramatically alter the practices used in animal agriculture.

Zoonotic Disease

The Centers for Disease Control, or CDC, reports that three out of four new emerging infectious diseases are zoonotic![2] A zoonotic disease is a disease that can be transmitted from animals to humans. They are caused by harmful germs like viruses, bacteria, fungi, and parasites.[3] These germs can cause various types of illnesses in people and animals, ranging from mild to severe to deadly.[4] It's estimated that 75% of viruses and 50% of bacteria known to cause disease in humans are zoonotic.[5]

---

[2] https://www.cdc.gov/onehealth/basics/zoonotic-diseases.html
[3] https://www.cdc.gov/onehealth/basics/zoonotic-diseases.html
[4] https://www.cdc.gov/onehealth/basics/zoonotic-diseases.html
[5] https://www.ncbi.nlm.nih.gov/pmc/articles/PMC3923154/

Zoonotic diseases don't just cause infections in humans, evidence suggests they may also be an underlying cause of certain types of cancer.[6] One example of this is the Bovine leukemia virus (BLV) infection. BLV is widespread in cattle globally and is present in many marketed beef and dairy products. BLV can be transferred to humans when they consume infected beef and dairy, and three case-controlled studies have found a significant association between BLV and breast cancer.[7] Zoonotic infections may also explain why meat and poultry workers have a greater risk of cancer death than any other worker groups.

Infectious Diseases and Animal Domestication

The first major spread of infectious diseases happened 10,000 -15,000 years ago when animals were first domesticated.[8] Author, doctor and professional speaker Michael Greger, MD, FACLM, points out there was another major spike during the industrial revolution when we brought animals to the barnyard.[9] And a third peak happened 30 years ago when we began to factory farm our animals. Medical observers

---

[6] https://www.ncbi.nlm.nih.gov/pmc/articles/PMC3923154/
[7] https://www.ncbi.nlm.nih.gov/pmc/articles/PMC3923154/
[8] https://www.ncbi.nlm.nih.gov/books/NBK45714/
[9] https://nutritionfacts.org/topics/zoonotic-disease/

call this time we are living in "The Age of Emerging Plagues," almost all of which come from animals.[10]

Animal Agriculture - A Breeding Ground for Infections

When it comes to the spread of zoonotic disease, factory farms are very problematic. Most animal products come from concentrated animal feeding operations, where the animals are locked up in dark, confined, crowded cages which provide the perfect breeding ground for infectious diseases. It's not unheard of to have 10 million birds in a single farm. They are fed unhealthy diets of corn, wheat, and soy grown in manure from animal poop and worse. At the time of slaughter, the feces of these animals concentrate billions of harmful bacteria like eColi and salmonella into our food and water supply.

I have examined "organic" chickens with or without antibiotic treatment loaded with bacteria before or after cooking. This is not to mention the contamination of viruses that are one thousand times smaller than bacteria, which are below the level of detection by most high-powered microscopes. These feedlot animals are raised in unnatural, stressful, and depraved conditions and this makes them extremely vulnerable to infections. These commercial chains allow pathogens

---

[10] https://nutritionfacts.org/topics/zoonotic-disease/

that were previously innocuous to rapidly spread, mutate, and become far more dangerous.[11]

Compounding the problem is the fact that animals that appear healthy carry germs that can make humans very sick.[12] One example of this is pigs, which are reservoirs of the Hepatitis E virus (HEV).[13] Research suggests this virus is in more than 10% of pig livers being sold across America.[14] Pigs infected with swine HEV are asymptomatic and appear clinically normal. With no way of identifying them, they end up at our grocery stores. The consumption of this meat, especially if undercooked, may result in HEV in humans.[15]

Please do not feel secure that by simply cooking your meat long enough you are safe. The fact is a number of studies show that many of these microbes survive extreme temperatures, 158 degrees Fahrenheit or 71 degrees Celsius for fairly long periods of over two hours. The high temperature still did not kill the bugs.[16]

Antibiotics will no longer protect us. The CDC reported over a quarter-million Americans are infected

[11] https://nutritionfacts.org/video/pandemics-history-prevention/

[12] https://www.cdc.gov/onehealth/basics/zoonotic-diseases.html

[13] https://www.ars.usda.gov/northeast-area/wyndmoor-pa/eastern-regional-research-center/residue-chemistry-and-predictive-microbiology-research/docs/pigs-people-and-hepatitis-e/

[14] https://nutritionfacts.org/topics/zoonotic-disease/

[15] https://academic.oup.com/ofid/article/6/9/ofz306/5523738

[16] Weese JS. Clostridium difficile in food-innocent bystander or serious threat? *Clin Microbiol Infect*. 2010;16:3-10

19 https://www.kansascity.com/news/virus/article242519791.html

with a type of colitis with painful, crampy diarrhea which mimics infection acquired from hospital workers. The infection actually came from the meat served in the hospital or from 42% of packaged meat products sold at three national grocery chain stores, killing thousands at a cost of One Billion Dollars a year! Alcohol-based hand sanitizers advertise they kill 99.9% of all germs but did not work either because residual spores are easily transmitted after touching raw or cooked meat.[17]

Animals Are Making Us Sick

If we all transitioned to a whole-foods, plant-based diet, we would dramatically reduce the spread and prevalence of infectious diseases. This nutritious way of eating would also help bolster our immune defenses so that harmful microbes don't get a chance to replicate and make us sick. Furthermore, we would dramatically lower our risk for most chronic diseases including cancer, heart disease, diabetes, and colon disease.

Additional Reasons to Give Up Meat

If Americans transitioned to a primarily plant-based diet, we would lower our reliance on sick-care and

---

[17] Jabbar U, Leischner J, Effectiveness of alcohol-based hand rubs for removal of Clostridium difficile spores from hands. *Infect Control Hosp Epidemiol.* 2010; 31(6):565-70

prescription drugs, and obesity would become less common. Our sex lives and sexual functioning would improve due to enhanced hormonal balance and healthier arteries that allow blood to flow to the pleasure organs. And we would increase our longevity and be protected from the 15 leading causes of death in the world.[18] We would also boost the health of our planet, as animal agriculture is a leading cause of global warming. We would put an end to the atrocious and inhumane treatment of animals in factory farms. A May 21, 2020 New York Times piece titled the *End of Meat*[19] by Jonathan Safran Foer came out talking about the fact that meats are readily available because we the taxpayers are allowing lawmakers "educated by lobbyists" to pay the feedlot industry huge subsidies to make hamburger, steak, chicken, or pork dishes affordable for all Americans to make us sicker.[20]

I know how important good recipes are because it took me over 15 years of searching the globe for incredibly tasty cuisines for us to assemble over 240 irresistible recipes. I truly believe consuming a plant based diet with the consumption of animal products reduced to no more than once or twice in a week or better yet per month may not only reduce the viral and

---

[18] https://jumdjournal.net/article/view/2892
[19] https://www.nytimes.com/2020/05/21/opinion/virus-meat-vegetarianism.html#click=https://t.co/GzgDiFOVkR
[20] https://www.nytimes.com/2020/05/21/opinion/virus-meat-vegetarianism.html#click=https://t.co/GzgDiFOVkR
**. https://delgadoprotocol.com/product/simply-healthy-ebook/

bacterial load sufficiently to end future lockdowns. This simple step could save millions of lives worldwide.

> *Coming up with delicious and healthy meal ideas can be tough when you first transition to a whole foods, plant based diet, because it's unfamiliar. I recommend you get a copy of the Simply Healthy Cookbook, as it's full of delicious, healthy, vegan, gluten-free recipes from around the world that your whole family will enjoy.*

A plant based diet rich in added blueberries, mushrooms, garlic, herbs, probiotics (pickles or cabbage), beans providing pre-biotics, raw fruits, and raw cruciferous vegetables can increase natural killer cells by double from 2 billion to over 4 billion cells to fight infections and disease.[21] Just 15 minutes of exercise will boost the immune system IgA (immunoglobulin, type A) antibodies in the saliva, moist mucosal area of the mouth, nostrils and eyes potentially by over 30%. This translates into far fewer respiratory infection and allergic symptoms.[22] [23]

---

[21] McAnulty LS, Effect of blueberries ingestion on natural killer cell counts, oxidative stress, and inflammation prior to and after 2.5 hour of running. *Appl Physiol Nutr Metab.* 2011;36(6): 976-84

[22] Berggren A, Randomised, double-blind and placebo-controlled study using new probiotic lactobacilli for strengthening the body immune defence against viral infections. *Eur J Nutr.* 2011;50(3):203-10.

[23] Jesenak M, Anti-allergic effect of pleuran(B-Glucan) in children with recurrent respiratory tract infection. *Phyto-ther Res.* 2014;28(3):471-4.

There are many cooking shows that feature sponsored animal-based recipes, however someday soon great cooks like Chef AJ who cooks without sugar, oil, salt, or processed foods will be properly featured. My son in-law Ramon is able to adapt animal-based to plant-based recipes while my son Chef Roman votes on recipes I have created on camera with thumbs up or down as I act as "Chef" Nick. It's hilarious because of my son's expressions and sincere comments. I love to cook or prepare my favorite raw plant-based dishes for my friends. When my family had an expecting child on the way or after birth, when there was no time to prepare meals, we ran an ad for a cook and provided the finalists with our original cookbook *Naturally Healthy*, created by Beth Delgado. Many of those recipes made the final cut for our best "Simply Healthy" dishes. See our favorite recipes voted by thousands of event attendees demonstrated at https://www.youtube.com/user/DelgadoVideo/search?query=recipes

Chapter 3:

Why the Adrenal Glands and Cortisol Are Essential to Immunity

Despite their miniature size, the adrenal glands play an indispensable role in your health. They are key modulators of immune function, responsible for secreting glucocorticoids and catecholamines which regulate immune cell activation, microbial proliferation, inflammation, and the expression of cytokines. The adrenal glands also help your body manage stress (which is a major immune system saboteur), and they produce DHEA, which plays a key role in immune competence. And finally, they release cortisol to keep inflammation in check, which is helpful because as we saw in the last chapter, the consequent cytokine storm and out-of-control inflammation are responsible for much of the damage that can occur when immune-compromised individuals contract certain pathogen infections.

Ongoing stress leads to elevated cortisol levels, and over time, can lead to exhausted adrenal glands, a cortisol deficiency, and chronic inflammation -- all of which compromise your immunity. Because stress is unavoidable in our modern world, many of us suffer with adrenal fatigue, and this makes us far more susceptible to contracting the virus.

We are actively doing ongoing research to tie in microscopic evaluations (images below are research only and not a diagnosis) as it relates to blood tests by reference labs such as lipid peroxidase along with exhaled breath with more oxidation. Over 50% of athletes and people are "mouth breathers" with a higher incidence to have respiratory disorders, asthma, sleep apnea and poor sleep habits which not only appears to increase oxidative stress, it may increase the risk of infections and shorten ones life.

Examples of Adrenal Dysfunction Under the Microscope

Oxidative stress shows up in the bloodstream from excess adrenaline overload

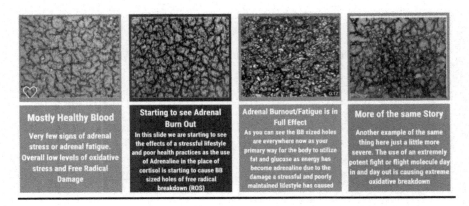

Mostly Healthy Blood	Starting to see Adrenal Burn Out	Adrenal Burnout/Fatigue is in Full Effect	More of the same Story
Very few signs of adrenal stress or adrenal fatigue. Overall low levels of oxidative stress and Free Radical Damage	In this slide we are starting to see the effects of a stressful lifestyle and poor health practices as the use of Adrenaline in the place of cortisol is starting to cause BB sized holes of free radical breakdown (ROS)	As you can see the BB sized holes are everywhere now as your primary way for the body to utilize fat and glucose as energy has become adrenaline due to the damage a stressful and poorly maintained lifestyle has caused	Another example of the same thing here just a little more severe. The use of an extremely potent fight or flight molecule day in and day out is causing extreme oxidative breakdown

Fortunately, there are several lifestyle modifications and herbs that you can use to boost adrenal function and help nourish them back to health which we will explore in Chapter 14.

Cortisol - The Immune System's Best Friend

Cortisol is arguably the most important hormone in the body. It provides amino acids, fatty acids, and blood sugar to all cells of the body while serving as the main trigger to the immune system. Cortisol produced by the adrenal glands may be the very remedy that works best in a crisis of severe infection, especially when used alongside adrenal support.

According to renowned endocrinologist William Jefferies, M.D., F.A.C.P., Clinical Professor of Internal Medicine, University of Virginia School of Medicine, inflammatory influenzas that have stricken past generations respond better to natural cortisol than synthetic corticosteroids and are best used at high dosages (up to two times above normal day to day physiologic levels) for several days during the onset and height of the infection.

In his book *Safe Uses of Cortisol*, Jefferies reports a study where sick patients were given bioidentical cortisol (not synthetic prednisone which comes with a plethora of risks and side-effects from long term use). "Clinical responses were striking. Within twenty-four hours all patients felt much better, and within forty-eight hours symptoms such as fever, malaise, and generalized aching had completely subsided, and they felt quite well. The initial dosage of cortisol was decreased after forty-eight hours and discontinued after six days of therapy. No relapses or complications occurred ..."

Medical Support "As a result of these findings, it was decided to treat patients with **acute influenza** in the same manner in which patients with **chronic adrenal insufficiency** were treated when they developed **acute respiratory infections**.

Cortisol, **20 mg** daily by mouth, **four times daily** before meals and at bedtime, was started. Patients were instructed to continue this dosage until they felt well, then decrease to **10 mg** 4 times daily for 2 days, then **5 mg** four times daily for two days then stop."

- **Safe Use of Cortisol** by William McK Jefferies MD

This approach is successful with other inflammatory diseases as well, including arthritis. Dr Jefferies states in Chapter 6 of his book that physiologic dosages in rheumatoid arthritis, autoimmunity, and adrenocortical deficiency recover with natural cortisol therapy (cortisone acetate or cortisol) and it can be taken indefinitely without harmful side effects. However, for the highest level of safety and protection, it is important to also support the body with DHEA cream and or bioidentical testosterone pellets to counterbalance the catabolic and anabolic effects.

It's important to note that hormonal intervention requires knowing how to conduct an orchestra for all instruments or functions of the body to be optimized. As such, it is advised that you work alongside a knowledgeable anti-aging doctor who understands that when working to build the immune system, you must first support adrenal health, then after weeks or even months, add anabolics (such as thyroid or androgens). If the doctor starts with anabolics in a person with weak adrenals, they will find their patients developing colds, flu or severe bronchitis, or pneumonia.

Chapter 4:

Methylation: A Vital Immune-Supporting Process

The only way a disease can take hold of a body is if multiple elements of the immune response are overcome.[24] There are numerous steps we need to take to optimize our immune systems, and one critical step is supporting methylation -- a process most people have never heard of, and yet without which, life would not exist.

What is Methylation?

Methylation is the process of transferring a methyl group (a single carbon atom attached to three hydrogen atoms), to another substance, altering its chemical structure and thereby changing it to something else. Methylation is a vital metabolic process that occurs in every single cell and organ of your body. Poor methylation is an extremely common and harmful

---

[24] https://www.pnas.org/content/115/5/E1012

condition that negatively affects almost every function of your body, and most people have no idea that they're suffering from it.[25]

How Poor Methylation Affects Your Virus Risk

Methylation is required for the DNA that is necessary for the production of new immune system helper cells such as T cells and B cells.[26]

Your DNA
And what you can do to change it for the better

Epigenetic modulation due to environmental factors (i.e., nutrition, xenobiotics, physical activity, stress, etc.) can actively influence gene expression in a cell- and tissue-specific manner.

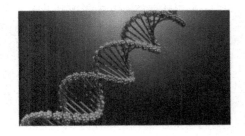

Methylation also plays a vital role in the suppression of viral DNA, and poor methylation allows the virus to hijack the cell and to replicate itself.[27] If you're methylating poorly, it hinders the immune response, making you more prone to infection

---

[25] https://www.bioceuticals.com.au/education/article/all-about-methylation-and-what-you-can-do-to-keep-yours-healthy
[26] https://www.nbwellness.com/library/methylation-health-disease/
[27] https://www.nbwellness.com/library/methylation-health-disease/

and increases the amount of time it takes for you to recover.

Another problem with poor methylation is that it increases your risk for chronic diseases that impair your ability to fight cardiovascular disease, cancer, and diabetes.[28] Your detoxification processes also become impaired, leading to the buildup of toxins in the body thus compromising your immune system.[29] And finally, poor methylation leads to inflammation, and several nutrient deficiencies, both of which further compromise immunity.[30]

Why Poor Methylation is So Common

Modern-day living subjects us to an overabundance of dietary and environmental toxins, often leading to poor methylation. Some common environmental toxins include plastics, mobile phones, laptops, radiation, cosmetics, cleaning and personal care products, pesticides, water pollutants, and industrial wastes. All of these toxins overwhelm the body and cause cellular damage which not only increases the body's need for methyl groups but also interferes with the body's production of methyl groups.[31] Methylation capabilities also decline with age and illness, and it is

[28] https://www.nbwellness.com/library/methylation-health-disease/
[29] https://www.nbwellness.com/library/methylation-health-disease/
[30] https://www.sciencedirect.com/science/article/pii/S2352304218300047
[31]

especially important to support this process if you are sick or elderly. Other factors that contribute to poor methylation include chronic stress, emotional trauma, and genetic errors.

How to Boost Methylation

Your diet heavily influences your ability to methylate. A whole foods-based diet that is low in sugar and fat, and high in vegetables is ideal. You should emphasize foods that contain methyl donors such as quinoa, beans, brown rice, chickpeas, beets, cruciferous vegetables, spinach, and other leafy greens. Choose organic whenever possible to reduce your intake of toxic herbicides and pesticides. And eliminate or vastly reduce your intake of vegetable oils, processed foods, caffeine, alcohol, refined sugars, and artificial additives and preservatives, because they are all highly toxic.

It is also vital that you exercise regularly. Exercise alters epigenetic methylation, directly influencing how your genes get expressed. Studies show notable positive changes occur in the genes within just three months of initiating a new exercise regime.[32] These changes in DNA methylation have been suggested to be the biological mechanism responsible for the many

---

32

http://journals.plos.org/plosgenetics/article?id=10.1371/journal.pgen.10035
72

beneficial effects of exercise.[33] Make sure to include high-intensity exercises in your workout regime; studies show they boost methylation.

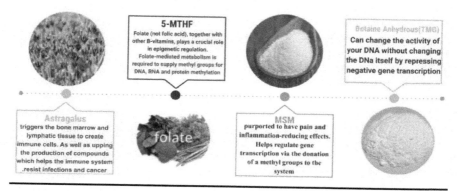

DNA **SUPER CHARGERS!**
Herbs rich in phytochemicals why you should eat them!

5-MTHF
Folate (not folic acid), together with other B-vitamins, plays a crucial role in epigenetic regulation. Folate-mediated metabolism is required to supply methyl groups for DNA, RNA and protein methylation

Betaine Anhydrous(TMG)
Can change the activity of your DNA without changing the DNa itself by repressing negative gene transcription

Astragalus
triggers the bone marrow and lymphatic tissue to create immune cells. As well as upping the production of compounds which helps the immune system resist infections and cancer

folate

MSM
purported to have pain and inflammation-reducing effects. Helps regulate gene transcription via the donation of a methyl groups to the system

Turbocharge Methylation with Methyl Donor Nutrients

Methyl donors are any substance that can transfer a methyl group to another substance, and they are required for optimal methylation. Methyl donor nutrients support and boost the methylation process.

Key methyl donor nutrients for enhancing methylation include:

---

[33]

http://journals.plos.org/plosgenetics/article?id=10.1371/journal.pgen.10035 72

- **MSM** (Methylsulfonylmethane) - Allows nutrients to flow more freely in the body and enhances detoxification.
- **TMG** (Trimethylglycine) - Assists in natural methylation.
- **PS** (Phosphatidylserine) - Essential for healthy brain function.
- **DMG** (Dimethylglycine) - Assists in cell metabolism and detoxification.

Foods to Eat to Optimize Your DNA

As methyl donors create CH3 molecule that breaks down rapidly while energy is produced to product DNA from byproducts of energy !

Flax, sunflower & Apricot Seeds
Flaxseed, have the potential to reverse obesity-associated gene expression via the regulation of DNA methylation and reduces the frequency of DNA damage that can lead to tumors

Black Beans & Astragalus
Have been shown in studies to down regulate glucose uptake genes directly related to cancer growth

Asparagus & Cyperus root
Filled with nutrients that play a crucial role in **epigenetic** regulation and cellular metabolism

Brazil Nuts & /CH3 methyl donor
The highest plant based source of Methionine the precursor to SAMe a potent methyl donor with many functions.

DNA Protector is a powerful methylation boosting product, formulated by leading anti-aging experts. It contains all of the key methyl donor nutrients outlined above as well as several B-vitamins which also act as methyl donors, and dramatically improving methylation.[34]* For more information on DNA protector and a full list of ingredients see the appendix, section one.

34

https://www.researchgate.net/publication/11222486_Diet_Methyl_Don ors_and_DNA_Methylation_Interactions_between_Dietary_Folate_Met hionine_and_Choline

Section 2:

Shocking Truths Revealed About the Immune System

Chapter 5:

How to Focus on the Positive Power of the Immune System rather than Fear of Disease

Studies show negative expectations can bring about adverse outcomes. It's a self-fulfilling prophecy and it is called the nocebo effect. The nocebo effect occurs when negative expectations increase the chances of having a negative outcome, and it is the opposite of the placebo effect. Don't fall victim to the nocebo effect - choose to be optimistic and focus on positive beliefs, natural solutions, and proactive actions, and you will be rewarded with healing and positive outcomes.

Humans have on average over 30,000 negative thoughts per day of which half are repeated the next day that creates stress which is the enemy of the immune system. As presented in *The Biology of Belief* by Bruce Lipton, stress is responsible for up to 90% of illnesses, including heart disease, cancer, and diabetes.[35] Stress can also cause people to eat poorly, consume more candy and junk food, and skip exercise, which further weakens immunity and increases disease risk.

Stress leads to depression and causes protective hormones such as testosterone, vitamin D3, and DHEA to decrease. Fear also causes the stress hormone adrenaline to be released in place of cortisol, and cortisol is the frontline hormone that protects us from disease.[36]

It is critical to understand that we also may choose our thoughts within a three-second window. Start practicing what we call the Three-Second Rule, which is count backwards 3, 2, 1 to first get into your conscious thinking mind, while pulling on a rubber band on your wrist, then say to yourself, "I will allow these negative thoughts to vanish and be nice to this person" as you reframe the sentence to a positive script. I use this three-second rule script sometimes as much as 20 times in a day! After several days, you will find the repeat negative is reduced and after a few months many of my students, according to my friend Darryl Wolf, find that over 95% of the negative thoughts are stopped in their tracks. Your world and how you view it, according the famous Endocrinologist Hans Selye, Author of *Stress without Disease*, believed that stress can

---

[35] https://www.brucelipton.com/books/biology-of-belief
[36] https://jeffreydachmd.com/wp-content/uploads/2013/03/Safe-uses-of-cortisol-Jefferies-William-McK-Charles-C-Thomas-2004.pdf

be useful when it is applied in a positive way to take action. Many heads of companies are "Type A" Personalities who allow time for mindfulness, rewards for tasks completed, and loving happy encounters with friends.

Stress can also be a time to make change and be more diligent about one's diet, supplements, exercise, and sleep. Every night I process my subconscious thoughts by listening to Neuro Reprogramming audio scripts with binaural beats in the theta (4 to 8 Hz) range. They are linked to relaxing REM sleep as well as meditative and creative states. When I have extremely stressful encounters during the day, I continue to remind myself to use the three-second rule, while at night I can process the information and make sense of the intellectual process to allow my subconscious mind to find solutions.

Most people with a healthy immune system and good adrenal function can recover from an infection rather rapidly so long as they're able to produce enough cortisol, ideally at least 40 mg a day or more if you are sick (we will explore how to increase cortisol levels in Section 3). There is a myth that high cortisol suppresses the body's defense system when in reality the opposite is true: cortisol is the front line of defense to help generate an immune response to fight infections and diseases.

The worst situations happen when a person suffers from dehydration or poor nutrition, both of which depress the person's ability to recover, especially in older individuals. In these instances, a complete shutdown of the immune system may occur to conserve the body's energy for running away from the perceived stressor, that proverbial "saber-toothed tiger." In fact, stress hormones are so effective at compromising the immune system that physicians therapeutically provide recipients of organ transplants with them to prevent their immune system from rejecting the foreign implant.

Foods To Eat to Improve White Blood Cell Quantity

Minerals and phytochemicals allow the immune system to mount a defense as needed

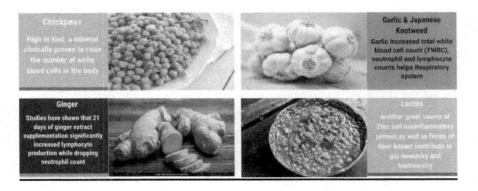

Chickpeas — High in zinc, a mineral clinically proven to raise the number of white blood cells in the body

Garlic & Japanese Knotweed — Garlic increased total white blood cell count (TWBC), neutrophil and lymphocyte counts helps Respiratory system

Ginger — Studies have shown that 21 days of ginger extract supplementation significantly increased lymphocyte production while dropping neutrophil count

Lentils — Another great source of Zinc and noninflammatory protein as well as forms of fiber known contribute to gut immunity and biodiversity

We must consider supporting older people with endocrinological intervention to bring their hormones and adrenal function to youthful levels. It is no coincidence that many of the longest living people in the world (such as in Okinawa) consume a mostly plant-based diet, have daily exercise built-into their lives, and use herbal rather than pharmaceutical medicines. These populations maintain more youthful levels of many protective hormones, including testosterone, DHEA, and healthy forms of estrogen, throughout their lives. In fact, one study found people who reached age 100 in these zones had levels of the aforementioned hormones that were equivalent to people who were 30 years younger in the USA.

The truth is you can drastically reduce your chances of getting sick, and promote quick and full recovery if you do, by optimizing your immune system.

We must understand that a healthy lifestyle is our greatest defense against any disease. The best thing you can do is to take steps to stay healthy with good nutrition, exercise, and nutraceuticals; and to support your adrenal glands and immune system by avoiding alcohol, sugar, oils and processed foods. It's also important that you avoid negative people and negative media, maintain loving relationships, improve hormone balance, and excrete toxins. When you follow the protocols in this book, you will have a powerful immune system, great health, and a long life.

No matter who you are and what your current state of health is, you will benefit from steering clear of the fear when you already know what to do by following your intuition, and supporting yourself in whatever way feels best to you. Bruce Lipton states: "Quantum physics, the most valid of all the sciences, emphasizes that our life experiences are founded in our consciousness."

Are you focused and conscious of disease . . . or of health, positive thoughts, and actions?

White Blood Cell Quantity SUPER CHARGERS!

And why you should eat them!

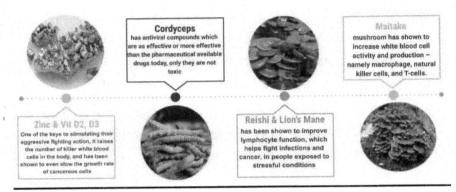

Cordyceps
has antiviral compounds which are as effective or more effective than the pharmaceutical available drugs today, only they are not toxic

Maitake
mushroom has shown to increase white blood cell activity and production – namely macrophage, natural killer cells, and T-cells.

Zinc & Vit D2, D3
One of the keys to stimulating their aggressive fighting action, it raises the number of killer white blood cells in the body, and has been shown to even slow the growth rate of cancerous cells

Reishi & Lion's Mane
has been shown to improve lymphocyte function, which helps fight infections and cancer, in people exposed to stressful conditions

Chapter 6:

Not All Pathogens Are Bad for You

Pathogens have a bad reputation. When people hear the word, most will automatically think of aggressive, infectious, invisible agents that make us sick. The two main pathogens, viruses and bacteria, are similar to bacteria in that some are harmful and disease-causing, while others are helpful and play a vital role in keeping us healthy. Many viral infections at a young age help to ensure the proper development of our immune systems.[37]

With each breath, we naturally breathe in over one hundred thousand various strains of viruses.[38] Many of these viruses are necessary to build our immune defenses, protect us from pathogenic viruses, and control harmful bacteria such as E.Coli and anthrax. Several strains are currently being studied for therapeutic use. For example, the herpes viruses (when latent) can help human natural killer cells identify

---

[37] https://phys.org/news/2019-08-viruses-nasty-health.html
[38] https://www.ncbi.nlm.nih.gov/pmc/articles/PMC4515362/

cancer cells and cells infected by other pathogenic viruses.[39] In the future, viruses like these could be modified and potentially used to target cancer cells.[40]

Another example of protective viruses are phages (or Bacteriophages). Phages are found in the mucous membrane lining of the reproductive, digestive, and respiratory tract. According to recent research, these phages are a part of our natural immune system, and they help protect us from invading bacteria.[41] Phages are currently being studied as a potential treatment for severe bacterial infections that are resistant to antibiotics.[42]

Humans have an average of 37 to 50 trillion human cells, about 39 trillion bacteria cells, and a massive 220 to 380 trillion virus cells.[43] Viruses are clearly not foreign to the body and we are not powerless against the pathogenic ones. Our immune system has evolved over millions of years to handle pathogens.

Your body produces over one million white blood cells every ten seconds, and B-Cells have over one billion combinations to address any invading microbe.

---

[39] https://phys.org/news/2019-08-viruses-nasty-health.html
[40] https://phys.org/news/2019-08-viruses-nasty-health.html
[41] https://www.pnas.org/content/110/26/10771
[42] https://www.theguardian.com/science/2019/may/08/teenager-recovers-from-near-death-in-world-first-gm-virus-treatment
[43] https://publichealth.wustl.edu/the-wonderful-world-of-virology/

Section 3:

How to Boost Immunity

Chapter 7:

Five Lifestyle Tips for Disease Prevention

Your risk of contracting a disease is largely in your hands. In this chapter, you will learn five easy and free lifestyle modifications that will boost your immune system and make you far less susceptible to disease.

#1 Get Enough Vitamin D

Almost half of all Americans are deficient in vitamin D because of a lack of adequate sun exposure, and this vitamin plays a vital role in the immune response. The sun converts dehydrocholesterol into Vitamin D3 under the skin, and when you don't get enough your immune system can't properly defend you from invading organisms and infections. The sun also boosts the release of powerful protective hormones such as testosterone and Luteinizing hormone, LH, which increases a whopping 67% from daily exposure to the sun.

If you live in a sunny climate, the best way to get your vitamin D is to expose your skin to sunlight. Even

15 minutes outdoors without sunglasses on will make a huge difference in the quality of your immune system. If daily sunlight exposure is not possible for you, you should consider supplementing with vitamin D to help your immune system. It's important that you choose a supplement in the natural form - D3 (cholecalciferol) as opposed to D2 (found in many cheaper supplements) because D3 is better absorbed, and studies show it is more effective at improving vitamin D status. Vitamin K2 used at 1 mg helps the Vitamin D3 to be absorbed into the bones rather than the arteries. It is best to combine some nuts, seeds or avocado when taking Vitamin D3 and Vitamin K2.

*Call our office 949-720-1554 and visit the appendix see Heart Insulin Stability, which provides 125 mcg or 5,000 IU Vitamin D3 per capsule and is shown to help boost circulating vitamin D levels. This combination is sure to improve your immune system to fight viruses. Be sure to have your blood levels tested about every 6 months until you reach ideal levels then monitor yearly to stay within the ideal range, not too low nor too high.

#2 Get Enough High-Quality Sleep

The importance of getting enough quality sleep cannot be overstated. During sleep, your body repairs itself, and your immune system releases protective proteins that play a critical role in protecting against bacterial and viral infections. And when you don't get enough quality sleep, your stress hormones increase, and infection-fighting antibodies and cells are reduced.

1. SLEEP & STRESS

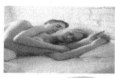

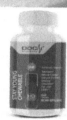

BETTER **SLEEP** required for strong immune system:

MELATONIN, NITRIC OXIDE, CBD, LFC scripts, Stay Young, Astragalus

Benefits of Quality sleep:

- 30% longer lifespan
- Improved cognition
- Fights dementia and Alzheimer's disease
- 50% less headaches
- Reduced cancer risk
- 34% reduced risk for **flu** or cold

One effective way to get better sleep is to turn the clock back by one full hour compared to your usual bedtime. Wake up without an alarm and use NLP Neuro Reprogramming audio scripts for amazing deep-delta rejuvenation sleep. Also try following sleep hygiene practices which include keeping electronics out of the bedroom, using a blue light filter on your laptop and phone in the evenings, keeping a regular sleep schedule, and sleeping in a cool, dark, and quiet environment. And if all else fails, consider CBD, melatonin, Stay Young tablets, nitric oxide therapy, or astragalus.

#3 Exercise Regularly

We all know that exercise is good for us in the long term - it helps regulate body weight, adds years to our lifespan, and reduces our risk for nearly every chronic disease. However, there is also an immediate benefit to your immune system. If you get your heart rate up, your circulation and the flow of oxygen and nutrients to your lungs and your body improves dramatically. The white blood cells and immunoglobulins which are used by the immune system to neutralize pathogens also improve, which helps your body find and destroy disease-causing microbes.

Exercise also helps to clear out congestion and flush pathogens out of the lungs and airways, reducing your chance of getting sick.[44] And it slows down the release of stress hormones such as adrenaline, which is beneficial because having lower stress hormones helps protect against illnesses. Finally, the brief rise in body temperature during and right after exercise helps ward off infections and prevents viruses from replicating in the body.

The Lymph System Benefits of Exercise

The lymph system plays a vital role in circulation and immunity. It acts like an inner highway that brings essential nutrients to all your cells and carries white blood cells throughout your body. Inactivity significantly restricts lymph flow and leads to a build-

---

[44] https://medlineplus.gov/ency/article/007165.htm

up of waste and toxins which play a role in inflammation and disease. Exercise, on the other hand, stimulates the flow of lymph fluid, so that the lymph can do its job of catching and destroying viruses, bacteria, and cellular waste, and eliminating infections from the body.

Which Exercise Is Best?

Although any exercise is better than no exercise, the best benefits come from exercises where you are breathing heavily during the entire period. Rebounding is particularly beneficial. Running or jumping on a bungee cord trampoline leads to approximately ten times more lymphatic flow through the body as compared to just walking, which helps to increase the efficiency of the immune system.

A balanced workout regime that includes strength training, stretching, rebounding and cardiovascular exercises is always best. If you are new to exercise, it is best to gradually build up in intensity, from walking to speed walking to running. Doing workouts with weights with little or no rest between sets is also going to dramatically improve your immune system. Choose a weight you can lift 50 times; if it's too heavy to do so, drop the amount of weight down until you can complete the set in one continuous nonstop fashion. See my video podcast blog for fun examples of exercise you can do at home or while traveling.

#4 Emphasize Love and Connection

We need to connect now more than ever. Use video calling apps to connect with your loved ones, family, and extended family daily -- this will contribute to healthy hormones and a stronger immune system. Sex and intimacy are also incredibly helpful (always protect yourself with a condom if you're not in a monogamous relationship). Cuddling, caressing, and lovemaking increase natural IGA antibodies that defend us from viruses. Hugs are also a great way to boost your immunity. Also do include the buildup of lovemaking tension to transmit your body's highest forms of energy to recover from potentially devastating illnesses. Read _Mastering Love, Sex & Intimacy_ now on Amazon for the best tips to harness the energy of love.

Reach out to old friends and make sure to demonstrate your love to your family and friends often. Feeling cared for boosts the immune system, and studies show it reduces the risk of contracting colds and viruses.[45] Those who have a loving support system also recover more quickly from illnesses, so make sure you reach out to all the elderly and sick in your life and let them know how much they mean to you.

---

[45] https://uthealthaustin.org/blog/health-benefits-of-love

#5 Reduce Stress and Focus on Positive Thoughts

Psychoimmunology:

Your psyche responses to the environment.

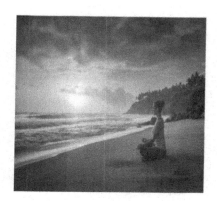

- If you're happy, exercising or spending time in the sun, your immune system works better
- If you worry or feel depressed, anxious or in a **fear state**, then your sympathetic nervous system gets triggered
- **Mediation** helps to turn off the sympathetic nervous system and turn on the parasympathetic nervous system.

Focus on happy empowering thoughts. Replace thoughts of unhappy childhood, trauma, or fear of disease with love. Be happy NOW. We have 60,000 thoughts/day, 50% are negative, and we move in the direction of our dominant thoughts.

You can use NLP audio scripts to guide the mind to happy consistent thoughts and actions. There are a variety of scripts for health and happiness at https://delgadoprotocol.com/product-category/hypnosis/. *If you listen daily upon waking in the morning when theta brain waves are highest, and again at bedtime when theta learning brain waves naturally increase again, it will reinforce your commitments to happiness and will begin to reprogram your subconscious mind for success within only seven days. Most of my clients find that their actions of eating healthier, exercising, and being mindful and joyful improve noticeably after two or three weeks.*

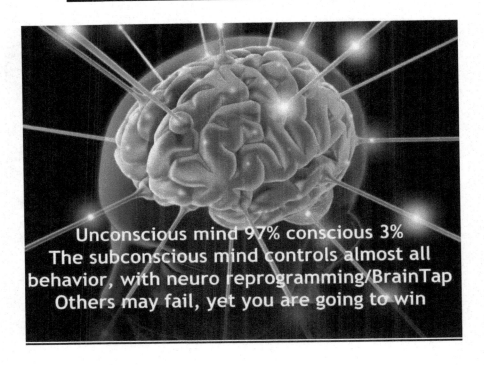

Unconscious mind 97% conscious 3%
The subconscious mind controls almost all behavior, with neuro reprogramming/BrainTap
Others may fail, yet you are going to win

It's essential that you limit stress. Taking precautions to arm yourself against disease is helpful but buying into the fear is not -- it activates the fight or flight response which reduces the immune system's ability to fight off infectious diseases. In other words, the more you stress, the more likely you are to get sick.

To help reduce stress, surround yourself with positive people and try engaging in at least one of the following stress-reducing activities daily: meditation, yoga, breathwork, Epsom salt baths, getting a massage, walks in nature, dancing, journaling, having sex, singing to music, or cuddling with a loved one.

Additional Lifestyle Tips for Boosting Immunity

Make sure to spend time in nature and laugh often. Live a mindful life with purpose, contribution, and personal development. Avoid smoking, drink alcohol in moderation or not at all, and maintain a healthy body weight. Perhaps most importantly of all, consume a whole foods plant-based diet (see the next chapter for specifics). Wash your hands regularly with soap for at least 20 seconds and avoid touching your face; this will help reduce your exposure to pathogens and thus lower the workload of your immune system.

The Jing Orb is also recommended, it acts as a body recharger. Like a Tesla car has to be recharged, our weak organs do as well, and the Jing Orb helps to strengthen the organs, to build immunity and fight infections. There is a growing body of evidence that by placing one's feet or hands or body into a tub of water with the orb generating energy vibrations, the water will transmit into your body and rejuvenate the immune system and organs by preventing unfolded proteins from accumulating. This therapy which I use for myself and my VIP clients may help autism,

Asperger's syndrome, Alzheimer's disease, cystic fibrosis, Gaucher's disease, and other neurodegenerative disorders. I also have an infrared relax sauna which I use for 35 minutes a day, while my feet remain cool in the Jing Orb bath.

Low-Level Laser Therapy can increase nitric oxide levels according to nitric oxide expert, Dr. Nathan Bryan, who I interviewed at the Anti-Aging Medicine conferences (A4M).[46] Bryan explains nitric oxide fills into white blood cells to concentrate its ability to fight microbes! We also use Grow Muscle Burn Fat powder at our clinic which contains organic beets rich in plant nitrates that convert into nitric oxide. This gas relaxes the blood vessels and increases oxygen to all the cells of the body.

Powerful Immune System:

(Alpha Stem, PEMF, Jing Orb and **Low Level Laser Therapy)**
PEMF – pulse electromagnetic frequency - enhanced immune system & blood flow to 74,000 miles microcirculation.
Cardiac, fitness, stress, sleep. **Far Infrared Relax Sauna** - increase core temperature.

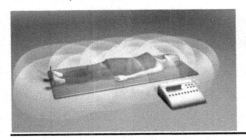

Benefits:
*Stronger immune system
*Autism – Aspergers
*Live longer free of toxins

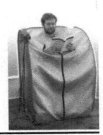

---

[46] https://drnathansbryan.com/

PEMF – pulse electromagnetic frequency – can also be used to enhance the immune system and blood flow. And an indoor air filter is highly recommended; studies show we can reduce the presence of viruses and bacteria in our homes to levels below that of outdoors. A couple of high-quality air filters to try include Fresh Air Everest (ionization requires no filter) and Oransi-HEPA Finn air purifier.

Chapter 8:

The Incredible Immune-Boosting Diet

Some places such as the blue zone -- Sardinia, Italy -- have far less sickness, a reflection of a healthy lifestyle that includes fresh outdoor air, exercise, quality sleep, loving connection, stress management, and perhaps most importantly of all - a healthy diet.

Every 10 seconds our bodies produce:

- 1 million new white blood cells (WBC) to sustain our immune system
- 20 million red blood cells (RBC) for circulation
- 30 million platelets to ensure proper clotting

The body also has older cells that need to be cleared away by the immune system. The right diet can support all these processes and rejuvenate our immune systems. The best diet for this and for warding off infectious and chronic diseases is a whole food, oil-free, sugar-free, plant-based diet. Eating this way will help reduce inflammation and oxidative stress and will ensure you get all the essential nutrients you need for optimal health and immunity. It will also increase oxygen delivery to the lungs and brain and provide you with plenty of protective phytochemicals.

Gut microbiome - Support with an anti-inflammatory, high fiber diet, that's organic and GMO-free, and contains unprocessed fats, resistant starches, and plant proteins.

*60-100 g fiber/day (Beans 14 g/c, Vegetables 4 g/c, fruit 3 g/c - 30% less calories, weight loss, water rich. Meat/Dairy 0 g fiber)

*Fiber acts like a magnet - Enterohepatic Circulation, reduces excess estrogen, cholesterol, and toxins.

LD50 Poison 100% Animals survive lethal dose, 50% die with no fiber

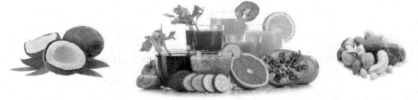

Phytochemicals: The Immune System Superstars

Plant foods contain protective phytochemicals that aren't found in animal products. Phytochemicals have an immune rejuvenation effect and support healthy immunity in a plethora of ways. First, they have potent antimicrobial properties to help protect us from mold, bacteria, and viruses.[47] Second, they help to reduce oxidative stress and inflammation, which improves overall health. Phytochemicals have also been found to stabilize the intestinal microbiota and reduce microbial toxic metabolites in the gut, and reduce stress on the

---

[47] https://www.ncbi.nlm.nih.gov/pmc/articles/PMC6066919/

immune system.[48] And finally, they increase the growth and spread (proliferation) of immune cells, they modulate cytokines, and they boost antibody production.[49]

Wild plants are typically superior to farmed ones because they evolved in stressful environments and as a result, they have more protective phytochemicals, nutrients and other beneficial compounds.[50] These nutrients grow without fertilizer; they can detoxify chemicals and survive extreme temperatures. One of the richest sources of phytochemicals is Himalayan tartary buckwheat. It has 100 times the phytochemical density of any other plant. We use tartary buckwheat, activated barley, medicinal mushrooms, and over 20 additional nutrient-rich ingredients in our supplements.

Consume Fruits and Vegetables Abundantly

The more fruits and vegetables you consume the better. Ideally, you should consume at least ten servings daily -- this will help detoxify your body and arm your immune system with essential nutrients and

---

[48] https://www.ncbi.nlm.nih.gov/pmc/articles/PMC6066919/
[49] https://www.ncbi.nlm.nih.gov/pmc/articles/PMC6066919/
[50]

https://www.researchgate.net/publication/235338623_Wild_edible_fruits_as_a_potential_source_of_phytochemicals_with_capacity_to_inhibit_lipid_peroxidation phytochemicals. Emphasize cruciferous vegetables because they contain DIM (Diindolylmethane) and I3C (Indole 3 carbinol) which are potent immune system stimulators that enhance viral clearance and help to detoxify harmful estrogens.[51] You may also want to remember the acronym GBOMB - greens, berries, onions, mushrooms, beans - and consume these immune-boosting foods frequently. And don't forget to use herbs and spices generously, especially turmeric, curcumin, cinnamon, cayenne pepper, and garlic.

Be sure to consume lots of fiber (aim for 60-100 grams/day). Fiber acts like a magnet and helps to clear out toxins, cholesterol, and excess estrogen. It also supports healthy bacteria in the gut, and helps generate molecular hydrogen, H2. Over 500 studies from Japan and around the world have found amazing therapeutic results from supporting healthy hydrogen levels. In addition to fiber, you can also boost hydrogen with H2 water generators.

Caffeine may also be a problem, since excess consumption tends to occur among people with adrenal burn out, and the terrapin acids in coffee further weaken the adrenal glands. There are a number of people who do not metabolize the ingredients in coffee, and I am one of them. If you take the amount of caffeine in two cups of coffee and you find yourself fatigued each day unless you drink more coffee, then

[51] https://www.ncbi.nlm.nih.gov/pmc/articles/PMC2387240/

give yourself a three-week break. After three weeks, provided you can last that long, see how you feel. During this time avoid coffee and if you need an energy boost, try consuming 64 oz of fresh vegetable juice daily instead.

You should also eliminate or vastly reduce your intake of oil, processed foods, and gluten - all three are inflammatory. And identify and eliminate any potential food intolerances to reduce gut inflammation. Limit your intake of alcohol to no more than one unit a day and eliminate stimulants, including sugar and caffeine.

The Three Worst Foods for Your Immune System

Below you will learn the three worst foods for your immune system. By eliminating these three foods from your diet, you'll reduce inflammation, fight aging and chronic disease, lose weight, bolster your sex drive, look younger and feel better!

Sugar

Every time you consume sugar it suppresses your immune system for at least a few hours, so if you eat it multiple times a day, your immune system may be perpetually operating at a distinct disadvantage. A high-sugar diet also leads to chronic inflammation and increases your risk for chronic diseases such as cardiovascular disease and diabetes; these diseases make illness more severe and reduce your body's ability to recover from it.[52] [53]

Sugar-containing foods are typically spiked with added processed fats and oils. This combination leads to high blood sugar levels and will desensitize your insulin. This can worsen the outcome of infections. A study published by the journal *Science Advances*, found chronically elevated blood sugar levels, as found in diabetics, promote a greater risk of cytokine storm which can lead to death.[54] This occurs because the metabolic pathway hexosamine biosynthesis allows for pathogens to go out of control.[55]

If you want optimal immunity, you need to cut out all types of sugar and sugar-containing foods, including the ones commonly considered 'healthy' such as honey, maple syrup, molasses, and cane sugar. Keep in mind that sugar is rarely consumed by itself. Often candies have very high amounts of fats combined with the sugars which further worsen the insulin, blood sugar levels, and depression of the immune system.

---

[52] https://www.ncbi.nlm.nih.gov/pubmed/29727694
[53] https://www.nationalgeographic.com/science/2020/03/these-underlying-conditions-make-virus-more-severe-and-they-are-surprisingly-common/
[54] https://advances.sciencemag.org/content/6/16/eaaz7086
[55] https://advances.sciencemag.org/content/6/16/eaaz7086

A recent poll showed that Americans' favorite candies are Reese's Peanut Butter Cups, Snickers, M&Ms, and Hershey Bars. All of these are extremely high in fat and sugar with dairy proteins, which actually damage white blood cells, as seen under the microscope. Here are the amounts of these harmful ingredients per serving of these "favorites":

- Reese's Peanut Butter Cup - 36% with 5 grams of fat, 22 grams of sugar, and over 220 calories per cup
- Snickers - 18% with 11 grams of fat, 12 grams of sugar, and over 280 calories
- M&M - 11% with 9 grams of fat, 31 grams of sugar, and 230 calories
- Hershey Bars - 6%, with 13 grams of fat, 21 grams of added sugar, and 220 calories

Each of the above also has over 5 mg of cholesterol per serving, which further paralyzes the immune system.

- Candies with "just sugar" were less often selected:
- Candy corn - 6% with 0 fat, 32 grams of sugar, and140 calories
- Skittles - 5% with 2 gram of fat, 43 grams of sugar, and 230 calories
- Starburst - 4% under 1 gram of fat, 4 grams of sugar, with 20 calories per piece

This doesn't even get into the issue of food coloring, additives, and chemicals that also dangerously damage the immune system. Ideally, your only source of sugar should be fruits and starchy vegetables. Remember, although fruit tastes sweet, they have special phytochemicals that will allow the blood sugar to remain stable making them safe to eat in large quantities.

Animal Protein

Just like sugar, a diet that is high in animal protein increases inflammation throughout your body and raises your risk for chronic diseases.[56] Animal products are also the primary carriers of highly infectious and contagious viruses, and they are high in estrogens, antibiotics and other toxins that overwhelm your liver and reduce your immunity. And if all that wasn't bad enough, consuming them alters the healthy, immune system-boosting gut bacteria, reducing their ability to fight off pathogens.[57] In fact, the US alone has millions of people dying monthly from causes related to an animal protein-based diet.

---

[56] https://www.frontiersin.org/articles/10.3389/fimmu.2019.00919/full

[57] https://www.npr.org/sections/thesalt/2013/12/10/250007042/chowing-down-on-meat-and-dairy-alters-gut-bacteria-a-lot-and-quickly

We need far less protein then we've been led to believe and can get all our needs met with a plant-based diet. Eliminating or vastly reducing your intake of animal products will not only support your gut health and immune system, but it will also help shave inches off your waistline, lower your cholesterol and blood pressure, reduce your medication requirements, enhance your skin health and add years to your life expectancy.[58] [59]

*For a variety of delicious, immune-boosting, anti-aging, plant-based recipes from different cuisines around the world, get a copy of the Simply Healthy Cookbook.

Oils and Other Separated Fats

Animal fats, and all fats that are separated from their fiber source, are bad for you. This includes all types of vegetable oils and all foods that contain oils (baked goods, chips, fried food, fast food, etc.). When you consume these fats, it causes your red blood cells (RBCs) to clump together for hours afterward, and RBCs are important modulators of the innate immune response.

---

[58] https://www.ncbi.nlm.nih.gov/pmc/articles/PMC5934425/
[59] https://www.ncbi.nlm.nih.gov/pmc/articles/PMC3662288/

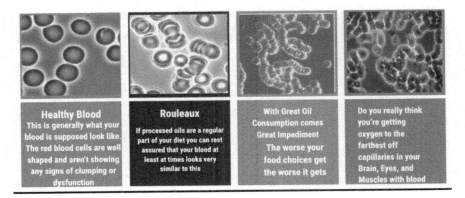

Examples of Bad Cardio Under the Microscope

Healthy blood flows freely while greasy thick blood flows slowly and clumps together reducing oxygen by over 30%

Healthy Blood	Rouleaux	With Great Oil Consumption comes Great Impediment	Do you really think you're getting
This is generally what your blood is supposed look like. The red blood cells are well shaped and aren't showing any signs of clumping or dysfunction	If processed oils are a regular part of your diet you can rest assured that your blood at least at times looks very similar to this	The worse your food choices get the worse it gets	oxygen to the farthest off capillaries in your Brain, Eyes, and Muscles with blood

Similar to sugar and animal proteins, a high-fat diet also leads to chronic inflammation and increased chronic disease risk. Saturated fats have been shown to "short-circuit" human immune cells.[60] This does not mean you should avoid all sources of fat; your body and brain need some healthy fats to thrive. But for optimal health and immunity, your diet should be low in processed fat, and the fat should come from healthy whole foods with their fiber intact, such as avocados, coconuts, olives, nuts, and seeds.

---

[60] https://www.cell.com/cell-reports/fulltext/S2211-1247(16)30174-7?_returnURL=https%3A%2F%2Flinkinghub.elsevier.com%2Fretrieve%2Fpii%2FS2211124716301747%3Fshowall%3Dtrue

Chapter 9:

How to Boost Adrenal Health, Cortisol Levels, and Immune Defenses

Earlier in the book you learned the essential role that the adrenal glands and cortisol play in supporting immunity and in both preventing and reversing the deadly cytokine storm. In this chapter you will learn how to optimize adrenal function, cortisol levels, and immune defenses with lifestyle medicine.

To maintain and restore adrenal and immune health it's important that you get enough high-quality sleep, exercise regularly (but be careful not to over-exert yourself), limit stress, and meditate or practice breathwork to help stabilize your nervous system. Following the dietary advice in the last chapter will also help to support your adrenal glands and immune system; however, when it comes to adrenal health specifically, it's important that you also make sure to eat something small every three hours, avoid overeating, and eliminate sugar, caffeine, and alcohol.

Foods to Avoid to Improve Adrenal Function

Destructive to those who have less ability to metabolize stimulants and junk food

Coffee

Nothing blows up already stressed adrenals worse than stimulants with coffee being one of the go to choices of man

Avoid it!!!

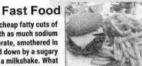

Energy Drinks

Nothing satisfies your body's energy and hormonal deficits like artificially sweetened, artificially colored, artificially flavored beverages with enough caffeine to cause a heart attack

Fast Food

Processed oil, cheap fatty cuts of meat infused with as much sodium as you can tolerate, smothered in cheese all chased down by a sugary beverage, and a milkshake. What could possibly go wrong?

Processed Food

GMO Fungus based Flavor enhancers, Artificial sweeteners and flavorings, laced with toxic preservatives all of which has never existed in the human diet before 100 years ago, put out for human consumption with no serious safety testing or oversight.

Because we live in such a high-stress and toxic world that constantly taxes our bodies, most of us would benefit from additional support. The following nutrients and herbs will nourish and support both the adrenal glands and the immune system. Many of them also function as natural antivirals and help to boost cortisol levels.

Nutrients and Herbs for Boosting Adrenal and Immune Function

Adrenal Cortex

Amla

Cinnamon Extract and Chromium

Dimethylglycine

Echinacea

Garlic Bulb Extract

Grapefruit Seed Extract (GSE)

Iodine
Licorice Root
Lomatium Root Powder
Vitamin C
Vitamin D
Zinc

1. Adrenal Cortex

Adrenal cortex (ideally derived from purified bovine sources from New Zealand) contains important adrenal hormones, including hydrocortisone (cortisol) which helps to support healthy cortisol levels in your body and reduce the workload of the adrenal glands. When combined with adrenal nourishing herbs, it helps to rebuild and rejuvenate tired adrenal glands, and restore them to health. Adrenal extract is beneficial to those with low adrenal function, fatigue, stress, lowered resistance to illness, severe allergies, asthma, skin conditions, and rheumatoid arthritis.

2. Amla

Amla is a potent antioxidant, anti-inflammatory, and anti-aging nutrient, and an excellent source of vitamin C, which is a well-known immunity booster. Because amla is a whole food, and not an artificial lab-created vitamin, the vitamin C it contains is more bioavailable, which means it is better absorbed and utilized by your body.

3. Cinnamon Extract and Chromium

Both cinnamon extract and chromium have been scientifically proven to help enhance insulin sensitivity and reduce blood sugar levels.[61] [62] This is beneficial because high blood sugar is known to weaken immune defenses. This explains why people with diabetes are more susceptible to developing infections and could also explain why people with diabetes are more likely to experience severe symptoms and complications.

4. Dimethylglycine

Dimethylglycine (DMG) helps the body regulate and manage stress and it improves the efficiency of cells throughout the body. It crosses the blood-brain barrier, enhancing mental capacity, supports liver and brain health, and acts as an immune system modulator. It also enhances the body's natural protection against bacterial, fungal, and viral diseases, and supports both methylations and the production of antibodies.[63]

---

[61] https://www.ncbi.nlm.nih.gov/pmc/articles/PMC3958529/
[62] https://www.ncbi.nlm.nih.gov/pubmed/15208835
[63] https://www.naturalmedicinejournal.com/blog/surprising-benefits-dmg-supplements

5. Echinacea

Echinacea increases the "non-specific" activity of the immune system. In other words, unlike a vaccine which is active only against a specific disease, echinacea stimulates the overall activity of the cells responsible for fighting all kinds of infections. Echinacea makes our own immune cells more efficient in attacking bacteria, viruses, and abnormal cells. It also improves the way that white blood cells fight against infective agents, lowers inflammation, and reduces symptoms, and speeds recovery.[64]

6. Garlic Bulb Extract

Garlic ranks highly among foods that help prevent disease, largely due to its high content of organosulfur compounds and antioxidant activity. Garlic boosts immunity, enhances immune cell numbers, and increases the activity of natural killer (NK) cells, which destroy invading organisms.

7. Grapefruit Seed Extract (GSE)

GSE has very high amounts of disease-fighting, free-radical eliminating antioxidants and phytonutrients

---

[64] https://www.ethicalnutrients.com.au/bodytalk/194-3-reasons-to-try-echinacea-this-cold-flu-season

called bioflavonoids. One of these powerful bioflavonoids, Hesperidin, is a well-known natural immune-system stimulator and booster. A recent study from *The Journal of Alternative and Complementary Medicine* found GSE was effective in killing over "800 bacterial and viral strains, 100 strains of fungus, and a large number of single and multi-celled parasites."[65] No other naturally-occurring antimicrobial can come close to these results.

8. Iodine

Iodine is a mineral that is essential for thyroid health, and a deficiency of it can lead to an under-functioning thyroid (hypothyroidism). Low thyroid levels accelerate aging, reduce metabolism, and increase the risk of infection. Iodine also has potent anti-viral properties and it helps the body to use oxygen. The World Health Organization states over 70% of adults are deficient in it, and these people would benefit from supplementation.[66] [67]

Worth noting, often thyroid levels show "normal" and appropriate to the reference range when tested, but

[65] 2. Graber CD, Goust JM, Glassman AD, et al. Immunomodulating properties of dimethylglycine in humans. J Infect Dis. 1981;143(1):101-5.

[66] https://www.urmc.rochester.edu/encyclopedia/content.aspx?contenttypeid=19&contentid=Iodine

[67] https://www.ncbi.nlm.nih.gov/pmc/articles/PMC7161480/

most doctors don't test T3 which is imperative to thyroid function, and many cases of hypothyroidism go undiagnosed. Some signs that you may be suffering with hypothyroidism include cold or swollen hands or feet, tendency to gain weight, low energy, low sex drive, mental fog, constipation, brittle nails, dry skin, and hair thinning.

> *To optimize iodine levels and support healthy thyroid function you can take Thyrodine. Thyrodine contains organic iodine and l-tyrosine which is another essential nutrient for the thyroid. Additional benefits of Thyrodine include healthy weight support, healthy metabolism, and radiation defense.*

9. Licorice Root

Licorice root has been used for centuries in Chinese Medicine to boost immunity, alleviate pain, tonify spleen and stomach, eliminate phlegm, and relieve coughing.[68] Researchers have identified several compounds in licorice root which demonstrate potent antimicrobial activities. They have found that glycyrrhizin (a naturally occurring compound in licorice) can significantly inhibit viral activity.[69] Licorice root is considered so effective at fighting off

[68] https://www.ncbi.nlm.nih.gov/pmc/articles/PMC4629407/
[69] https://www.ncbi.nlm.nih.gov/pmc/articles/PMC4629407/

infections that some researchers are proposing we use it to create affordable medicines to combat diseases in third-world countries. Licorice is additionally beneficial because studies show the glycyrrhetinic acid it contains helps maintain healthy cortisol levels by inhibiting the enzymes that break it down. [70] [71]

10. Lomatium Root Powder

This robust desert parsley has been extensively studied for immune health benefits and antioxidant abilities and has been used for centuries in traditional medicine to treat influenza and other respiratory tract infections.[72] Lomatium helps calm down inflammation, reduces viral load, and protects lungs against injury from colds and flu.

A recent study published in the *AARM Journal* found that lomatium helps reduce morbidity and mortality of influenza viruses by lowering levels of the cytokine CXCL10. This is beneficial because high levels of CXCL10 are associated with the initiation and progression of infectious diseases, and can lead to out of control inflammation and immune dysfunction.[73]

---

[70] https://www.ncbi.nlm.nih.gov/pubmed/21184804
[71] https://www.mdpi.com/2218-273X/10/3/352/htm
[72] https://restorativemedicine.org/journal/lomatium-dissectum-inhibits-secretion-of-cxcl10-a-chemokine-associated-with-poor-prognosis-in-highly-pathogenic-influenza-a-infection/
[73] https://www.ncbi.nlm.nih.gov/pmc/articles/PMC3203691/

> *Adrenal Immune Support is a clinically formulated nutraceutical that contains adrenal cortex and all of the above herbs and nutrients (minus iodine) as well as several additional adrenal optimizing, immune boosting, and energy enhancing herbs. It provides naturally occurring cortisol and leads to an immediate boost in adrenal function and immunity. *For more information and recommended dosages of Adrenal Immune Support for the prevention and quick reversal of infections, see section one of the appendix.*

11. Vitamin C

Vitamin C is well known as an immune system booster, and it supports lymphocytes, neutrophils, and other important regulators of the immune system. For a deeper exploration of Vitamin C, dosage recommendations, and how it may help prevent infections and hasten recovery see the appendix.

12. Vitamin D

When you don't get enough vitamin D the innate and adaptive immune responses are weakened and your immune system can't properly defend you from invading organisms and infections. A deficiency is also associated with increased autoimmune disorders.[74]

---

[74] https://www.ncbi.nlm.nih.gov/pmc/articles/PMC3166406/

13. Zinc

Zinc supports the production of several immune system helper cells including T-cells, neutrophils, and natural killer cells, and if you are deficient in it, you will be more susceptible to infections.[75] According to Science Daily recent research shows, "Zinc helps control infections by gently tapping the brakes on the immune response in a way that prevents out-of-control inflammation that can be damaging and even deadly."[76] Studies have also found zinc supplements help reduce the duration of infections.[77]

Insulin Heart Stability: If you want to support your immune system with a supplement that contains a blend of immune boosting nutrients, including licorice root, amla, cinnamon, chromium, probiotics, and vitamin D3 and zinc in their most bioavailable forms, try Insulin Heart Stability.

---

[75] https://www.ncbi.nlm.nih.gov/pubmed/9701160
[76] https://www.sciencedaily.com/releases/2013/02/130207131344.htm
[77] https://www.ncbi.nlm.nih.gov/pmc/articles/PMC3273967/

Chapter 10:

The Importance of Detoxification

We are exposed to toxins 24-7; they are in our water, our food, our cars, our homes, and our personal care products. Your liver is your primary detoxification organ, and it can easily become overwhelmed by the constant onslaught of toxins. When it does, toxins build up in your body, and your immune function can become severely compromised as a result. Moreover, our livers create immune system factors that can fight against infections. When our livers are healthy and strong, they are able to mount a rapid and robust immune response and detect, capture, and clear bacteria, viruses, and macromolecules. When they are functioning sub-optimally, we become much more susceptible to contracting diseases.[78]

To optimize liver health, eat a high-fiber, low-fat, whole foods-based diet and consume the following liver cleansing superfoods: cruciferous vegetables, citrus, beetroot, turmeric, ginger, wasabi, and garlic. It's also important that you vastly reduce your intake of, or

---

[78] https://www.ncbi.nlm.nih.gov/pubmed/29328785

eliminate, sugar, caffeine, processed and packaged foods, oils, and animal products. All the aforementioned foods place an unnecessary burden on your liver and can make it harder for your liver to do its job. Over time they also lead to inflammation, which in turn could cause scarring of the liver (cirrhosis). Finally, exercise regularly -- it helps to burn triglycerides for fuel, which reduces liver fat.

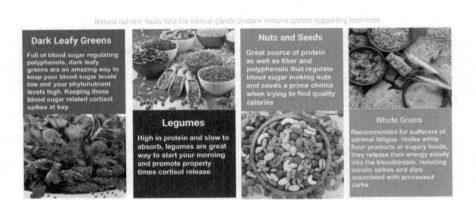

Foods to Eat to Boost Adrenal Function

Natural nutrient foods help the adrenal glands produce immune system supporting hormones

Dark Leafy Greens
Full of blood sugar regulating polyphenols, dark leafy greens are an amazing way to keep your blood sugar levels low and your phytonutrient levels high. Keeping those blood sugar related cortisol spikes at bay.

Nuts and Seeds
Great source of protein as well as fiber and polyphenols that regulate blood sugar making nuts and seeds a prime choice when trying to find quality calories

Legumes
High in protein and slow to absorb, legumes are great way to start your morning and promote properly times cortisol release

Whole Grains
Recommended for sufferers of adrenal fatigue. Unlike white flour products or sugary foods, they release their energy slowly into the bloodstream, reducing insulin spikes and dips associated with processed carbs

To reduce your chemical exposure, buy a water filter for your tap and shower, and consume at least eight glasses of water a day to help flush out toxins. Also, use organic personal care and cleaning products with natural ingredients, and exercise to the point of sweating at least three times a week. If possible, you should also avoid recreational, over the counter, and pharmaceutical drugs. If you have a chronic health condition or are currently on prescription medications, consider working with an anti-aging MD, DO, DC or Naturopathic doctor to support your health and minimize your medication requirements (but never do this on your own because changes or suddenly stopping medications can be dangerous or deadly!).

Another major source of toxins is alcohol. Individuals who consume alcohol regularly have decreased liver function, increased levels of immunoglobulins in their bloodstream (indicating an autoimmune response), and a greatly impaired immune system. Even if you only consume alcohol occasionally, it adds to your toxic load and places an unnecessary burden on your liver and immune system. Belarus has the highest alcohol consumption in the world, and people in France drink as little as one glass of wine every day yet they have the highest death rate from cirrhosis of the liver!

If you choose to drink alcohol in spite of this knowledge, it is recommended that you limit your intake to one serving. Also choose pear cider or apple cider beer which is free of yeast. Ideally, you should drink less than four standardized servings of wine, beer, and liquor per month. And avoid cocktails, liqueurs and soda mixed beverages because they are loaded with sugar, which is almost as harmful to your health and immunity as alcohol.

Defend Yourself with Herbs

There are several herbs that can help support your liver so it can properly eliminate toxins and excess hormones, reduce inflammation, and mount a strong immune response, including:

Turmeric

The active ingredient in turmeric -- curcumin -- has potent anti-inflammatory properties. It is also a potent immunomodulatory agent that can modulate the activation of numerous immune system helper cells, including T cells, B cells, macrophages, neutrophils, natural killer cells, and dendritic cells. Due in part to its ability to modulate the immune system, it has been found helpful in the management of arthritis, allergies, asthma, atherosclerosis, heart disease, Alzheimer's disease, diabetes, and cancer.

Ginger

Ginger is a potent antioxidant. Research shows it supports healthy immunity and can help treat a wide range of diseases via immuno-nutrition and anti-inflammatory responses. Ginger has also been found to play a protective role in gastric ailments such as ulcers, vomiting, nausea, dyspepsia, stomach aches, spasms, and gastrointestinal cancer.

Wasabi Root Powder

Current research is focused on the isothiocyanates (ITCs) that provide the majority of activity. Many scientists have concentrated on 6-MITC, of which Wasabia japonica contains a high concentration. There is now evidence showing that wasabi and its ITCs help protect against cancer, reduce diarrhea (Nakayama et al., 1998); protect nephrons in diabetes patients (Fukuchi et al., 2004); act as potent antioxidants (Gao et al., 2001; Lee et al., n.d.); and provide immune modulation (Manesh and Kuttan, 2003).

Liver Accel: *Liver Accel is a clinically formulated supplement that contains turmeric, ginger, wasabi, milk thistle and additional antioxidant dense super herbs that support liver function, fight inflammation, and bolster the immune system. *For a complete list of ingredients and benefits see appendix, section one.*

Milk Thistle

Milk thistle is one of the most commonly used herbs for supporting liver health. It can help reverse damage caused to the liver and it promotes the regeneration of new, healthy liver cells.[79] It also helps promote healthy

---

[79] https://www.ncbi.nlm.nih.gov/books/NBK11896/

cholesterol and insulin levels, reduces inflammation, and may help strengthen the immune response.[80]

---

[80] https://www.ncbi.nlm.nih.gov/books/NBK11896/

Chapter 11:

Four Hormones to Become Immune to Pathogens

As demonstrated in earlier chapters, cortisol is a vital hormone for the prevention and healing of diseases, but it's not the only hormone. In this chapter, we will explore four additional hormones that need to be optimized in order to minimize your risk for infectious diseases.

Insulin

Insulin and insulin sensitivity help prevent high blood sugar which is known to weaken immune defenses and increase inflammation. Recent research has also revealed immune cells are regulated by metabolic signals from insulin. Scientists from Toronto General Hospital identified a specific insulin signaling pathway that, when activated, increases the response of

T-cells in the immune system, which are white blood cells that play a key role in immunity.[81]

According to Senior Author, Dr. Winer: "T-Cells need more signals to boost their activation after they encounter a foreign invader . . . the insulin receptor or signaling molecule is like a second push to the immune system to ensure that it can fight off the infection with the best possible weapons it has."[82] The researchers believe this link is the explanation for why obese insulin-resistance individuals have weakened immune responses, and increased susceptibility to developing severe infections. This could also explain why people with diabetes are more likely to experience severe symptoms and complications when ill.

So how can this knowledge help protect you? If you want to optimize your immune system, you need to optimize insulin sensitivity and regulate your blood sugar levels. In order to do so, you should consume a high-fiber plant-based diet prepared without oils with lots of colorful fruits and vegetables, citrus, herbs and spices; and eat something small every three hours based on intuitive eating as you feel weak or hungry. Be sure to get more sleep, exercise regularly, and reduce stress. If you struggle with sticking to a healthy

---

[81]
https://www.uhn.ca/corporate/News/PressReleases/Pages/Insulin_give s_an_extra_boost_to_the_immune_system.aspx

[82]
https://www.uhn.ca/corporate/News/PressReleases/Pages/Insulin_give s_an_extra_boost_to_the_immune_system.aspx

eating plan or exercise regime get the LFC hypnosis tracks. Listen to them daily, and it will program your subconscious mind and eliminate the struggle.

Worth noting, some of my clients, even on a "healthy" plant-based diet, have had difficulty stabilizing their insulin levels and reducing lipids. These individuals did not respond even after more careful enforcement of dietary habits which included 24-hour food recall and a FitBit to record pictures of their food for a more accurate food record.

When these clients were instructed to take a focused supplement that included the insulin- stabilizing, lipid-reducing nutrients chromium, zinc, Vitamin D, policosanol, berberine, lycopene and bergamote, they responded remarkably well. Even those who had liver issues, genetic challenges, or less than ideal eating habits responded to this synergistic blend of nutrients. Their insulin stabilized, there was a reduction in LDL (the bad cholesterol), and there were improvements in the good HDL cholesterol levels.

Testosterone

Testosterone replacement therapy has been used for over 70 years in both men and women to treat symptoms and various diseases. It has immune-modulating properties, and current in vitro research suggests it may increase the expression of anti-inflammatory cytokines and reduce the expression of pro-inflammatory cytokines, both of which help to reduce inflammation throughout the body. This is beneficial to immunity because chronic inflammation leads to autoimmunity and several chronic diseases which can negatively affect your immune system.

Studies also show bioidentical testosterone replacement therapy lowers total cholesterol, and the combination of reducing inflammation and cholesterol bolsters cardiovascular health. This is helpful when it comes to viruses because cardiovascular disease is linked to severe symptoms and a higher risk of death. The heart is able to beat continuously awake or asleep partly because the heart has more testosterone receptor sites than any organ in the body!

A more affordable and yet still highly effective option can be found in nutraceutical creams and herbal testosterone boosting supplements, such as TestroGenesis Cream, Testro Genin cream, or Testro Plus capsules. For more information on these all-natural testosterone-boosting formulas and their benefits and uses, see the Appendix, section one.

Avoid conventional synthetic injectable testosterone replacement therapy (TRT) as it is associated with many harmful and troublesome side-effects and there are safe and effective alternatives available. BHRT is a bioidentical hormone replacement, yet one problem with compounded testosterone cream is it rarely has any herbs added to reduce conversion to estrogen, and worse, these compound pharmacies use a base cream loaded with chemicals.

Options for Safely Boosting Testosterone

The most expensive option is testosterone pellets which are implanted under the skin. Because they are bioidentical and mimic the body's own testosterone release system, they are safe and have few side effects. However, they are safest and most effective when combined with extra strength DIM products such as DIM 259, Estroblock Pro, or DHT Block along with Liv D-tox.

Sex-Hormone-Binding-Globulin (SHBG)

Sex-hormone-binding-globulin, or SHBG, is a protein produced by the liver that binds to and eliminates excess sex hormones from the body. SHBG protects you from colds and flu by binding to excess prolactin, thereby preventing prolactin levels from rising too high. This is helpful because high levels of prolactin increase pro-inflammatory immune responses and can lead to immune system dysfunctions.[83] [84] [85] These immune dysfunctions can make you more susceptible to infectious diseases.

To optimize SHBG levels it is important that you eliminate or vastly reduce your intake of fish, chicken, eggs, pork, and meat. Replace animal proteins with plant-based protein such as beans, rice, potatoes, and yams. Try to consume 15 servings of fruits and vegetables per day. This will help nutrify your skin and the water and fiber will help flush out toxins and excess hormones. It will also accelerate weight loss, which is beneficial because excess body weight lowers SHBG.

To meet the 15 recommended servings a day, try consuming vegetable casseroles made in a crockpot with several spices, as well as large soups and salads with dairy-free dressings. Finally, consume a low-fat diet and avoid all oils (olive oil, coconut, butter, etc). This will further increase SHBG levels, reduce prolactin, and decrease oil production in the skin.

Human Growth Hormone

Human growth hormone (HGH) influences the regeneration of every cell in the body, and this includes crucial immune cells. It has been found to promote the growth of the thymus, a gland that's responsible for the production of T-cells. It also stimulates the production

[83] https://www.ncbi.nlm.nih.gov/pubmed/11182231
[84] https://www.ncbi.nlm.nih.gov/pubmed/15319167
[85] https://www.ncbi.nlm.nih.gov/pubmed/11182231

of T-cells and B-cells, both of which play an essential role in immunity. Plus, it stimulates the synthesis of immunoglobulins, which are proteins made by the immune system to fight viruses and other antigens. And finally, it modulates cytokine response, which is beneficial because cytokines signal T cells, B cells, and other helper cells to move towards sites of inflammation, infection, and trauma.

To boost HGH, reduce your sugar intake, consume a low processed-fat diet, partake in high-intensity exercise, and get high-quality sleep by implementing sleep hygiene methods. Cellular aging and fasting expert, Dr. Volter Longo PhD, also recommends short intermittent fasts where you skip meals past 8 p.m. and don't eat until the next day starting at 8 a.m.

Chapter 12:

Rejuvenate Your Immune System with Peptide and Mitochondria Support

Rejuvenate the Immune System

Rejuvenating the immune system is something that people of all ages can benefit from. However, it is especially imperative for those over the age of 30 because immune function naturally declines with age. It's also vital for individuals of any age who have a chronic disease, who habitually use drugs or abuse alcohol, or who tend to get sick often. Two advanced methods for rejuvenating the immune system include peptide therapy and mitochondria support.

Peptides

Peptides are small proteins that are made up of short chains of amino acids. There are several thousands of them, and they play varying roles in the body. Peptide therapy is an exciting new frontier in medicine that can be used to safely reverse disease, boost immunity, enhance lovemaking, and decelerate the aging process.

For over 30 years it has been known that peptides are critical factors in mobilizing the immune system against foreign invaders including viruses, bacteria, and fungi.[86] They have been found helpful in managing autoimmune and immunodeficiency disorders.[87] [88] They've also been found to help repair leaky gut which is a major contributing factor to autoimmune diseases and poor immunity.[89]

Some promising peptides that are currently being studied and used for immune support, as well as warding off aging and disease and optimizing performance include:

- BP157- Has a regenerative effect on the entire body; and has been found to accelerate healing. [90]
- Beta thymosin - Naturally occurring and found in all tissues and cells (except red blood cells). This peptide demonstrates a wide range of regenerative activities.[91] It stimulates

---

[86] https://www.nature.com/articles/nchembio.1409
[87] https://www.ncbi.nlm.nih.gov/pmc/articles/PMC154453/
[88] https://www.ncbi.nlm.nih.gov/pmc/articles/PMC140873/
[89] https://agemed.org/wp-content/uploads/MARTINEZ-Peptides-for-Autoimmune-Disease.pdf
[90] https://pubmed.ncbi.nlm.nih.gov/21030672/
[91] https://www.sciencedirect.com/topics/biochemistry-genetics-and-molecular-biology/thymosin-beta-4

the production of T-cells, which play an important role in immunity. It appears to protect and regenerate injured and damaged tissue. It is also currently being investigated as a potential therapy for the treatment of immunocompromised disorder and influenza.[92]

- GHRP 6 - Stimulates the secretion of growth hormones.[93]

- IGF1 - Has nerve regenerative factors and capabilities, helps with muscle regeneration, supports skeletal and cardiovascular health.[94] Also plays a vital role in DNA and RNA synthesis; cell division, immune system function, and red blood cell production.[95]

- PT141 - Improves libido, pleasure, fantasy, performance, and orgasmic intensity. Can yield a huge improvement in sexual dysfunction in both genders.

- CJC1295 - Increases growth hormones and is used for anti-aging purposes and inflammatory conditions.[96]

- HGH (Human Growth Hormone) - Of the eight critical hormones that decline with age,

[92] https://www.sciencedirect.com/topics/biochemistry-genetics-and-molecular-biology/thymosin-beta-4
[93] https://pubmed.ncbi.nlm.nih.gov/7772238/
[94] https://www.ncbi.nlm.nih.gov/pmc/articles/PMC6367275/
[95] https://www.ncbi.nlm.nih.gov/pmc/articles/PMC6367275/
[96] https://pubmed.ncbi.nlm.nih.gov/16352683/

this peptide hormone is the most important. It's essential for slowing the aging process and if levels are restored past the age of thirty-five, it produces some rather amazing age reversal results. It also stimulates T and B cell proliferation and immunoglobulin synthesis.[97]

Safety and Precautions

Peptides are available as injections and in supplement form, and when taken orally they are extremely safe. There aren't many limitations or risks associated with peptide nutraceuticals, so long as you purchase them from a reputable company and take them as directed. However, I do recommend you start at the minimum suggested dosage, monitor results and effects, and adjust accordingly.

The Safe, All-Natural Peptide Booster

Amino acids are the building blocks of peptides. Some beneficial amino acids that you can supplement with to support peptide synthesis include l-arginine, l-glutamine, l-glycine, l-lysine, l-ornithine, and l-tyrosine.

---

[97]

https://www.researchgate.net/publication/7329964_Effect_of_growth_hormone_GH_on_the_immune_system

*If you want to start receiving the benefits of peptides immediately and to have the comfort of knowing what you are taking is safe and effective, then get Grow Muscle, Burn Fat. This proprietary anti-aging formula contains bioavailable protein peptides (vegan) and amino acids (including all those mentioned above) to release HGH and other healing growth factors. Experience a stronger immune system, reduced signs of aging, explosive energy, improved sports performance and stamina, quicker recovery time, rejuvenating sleep, enhanced lovemaking, and renewed cellular and organ health. *See appendix, section one for the full ingredients label and benefits.*

Mitochondria

Everyone is born with trillions of mitochondria, the multifunctional life-sustaining organelle that helps your body run. They dictate the fate of cells and when they aren't functioning properly, it impacts every cell in your body. In immune cells, the mitochondria can regulate cell development, activation, proliferation, differentiation, and death. Mitochondria also orchestrate the immune system by modulating both metabolic and physiologic states in different types of immune cells.

A large body of evidence indicates that mitochondria play a vital role in innate immunity, and most common aging-related diseases are caused, at least in-part by mitochondrial dysfunction. [98]It is hypothesized that the decline in mitochondrial function that naturally occurs with age is responsible for the elderly's greater susceptibility to viral infections, chronic inflammation, and an inability to recover from illnesses[99]

Aging, genetics, a toxic diet or lifestyle, hidden infections; heart disease, cancer, dementia and several other chronic diseases can all lead to mitochondrial dysfunction.[100] Now for the good news - you can increase the number and function of your mitochondria substantially. No matter what card you may have been dealt, or how old you are, you have the power to turn things around and support your immune system in doing it's job by implementing the below strategies.

Eat the Right Diet

The biggest determiner of your mitochondrial function is your diet. When you eat lots of refined, processed foods, sugar, white processed grains, fried foods, vegetable oils, dairy, factory farmed meat and other inflammatory foods, or simply eat too much calorically dense food, you overload your

---

[98] https://www.ncbi.nlm.nih.gov/pmc/articles/PMC6627182/
[99] https://www.ncbi.nlm.nih.gov/pmc/articles/PMC6627182/
[100] https://my.clevelandclinic.org/health/diseases/15612-mitochondrial-diseases

mitochondria and damage them. Avoid these foods and follow the dietary guidelines in Chapter 13 to support your mitochondria.

CVAC - The Remarkable Peak Fitness and Antiaging Process

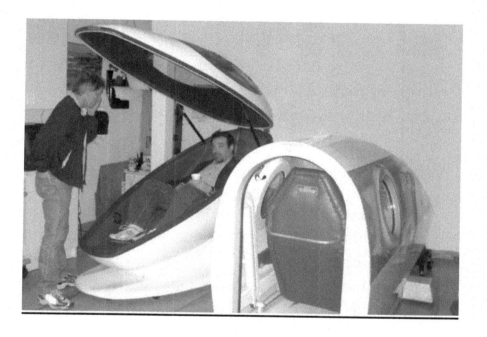

Research shows high intensity interval training (HIIT), where you go all-out for 30 to 60 seconds, slow down for a couple minutes, and repeat, is the most effective type of exercise for improving mitochondrial function. I include cyclic variations in altitude conditioning called CVAC, where I sit in a pod for 20-minute sessions to increase EPO building red blood cell volume for increased oxygen delivery, increased mitochondria, and more rapid recovery after exercise. A regular practice will lead to new, improved mitochondria.[101]

The Cyclic Variations in Adaptive Conditioning Process, or CVAC process offers a revolutionary way to achieve peak fitness, reverse aging, rejuvenate the organs, and protect against disease. Although many in-the-know professional athletes use it to uplevel their games, it is not well known by the general public, which is a shame because the benefits are both numerous and remarkable. Read on to discover what CVAC is, how it works, and how it can benefit you.

What It Does

The CVAC is a human-sized pod that you sit inside, typically for 20 minutes at a time. It steadily draws air out to create a low-pressure environment and sends filtered air in to create changes in air pressure and density. The body experiences similar challenges as it does when you climb in altitude or partake in high-altitude conditioning. A state of mild hypoxia (oxygen debt) occurs and the body responds by increasing red blood cells which supports oxygenation of the body.

CVAC Versus Altitude Training

---

[101] https://www.sciencedaily.com/releases/2017/03/170307155214.htm

What sets CVAC apart from altitude training is the fact that the change in air pressure isn't constant; it varies throughout the session, simulating increases and decreases in altitude. The challenge of continually adapting to different simulated altitudes leads to many additional benefits and because the amount of time spent in each altitude is so short, the maladies associated with altitude sickness do not occur. In fact, the CVAC has an incredibly high safety record. The total documented number of CVAC sessions is 334,718 and according to data from CVAC president Allen Ruszkowski there have been no significant adverse events reported in any of them.

CVAC Benefits

According to Allen, "CVAC's unique potential to improve tissue oxygenation, enhance lymph, organ and glandular function, as well as reduce inflammation suggests that CVAC's use in therapeutic applications could be very broad once we obtain the necessary data and approvals." During the CVAC Process the waves of tension and resolution gives the lymphatic system a 'touchless massage,' which facilitates the removal of metabolic waste products.

CVAC also gives the mitochondria a workout and increases their strength and efficiency. The mitochondria are the energy-producing parts or "powerhouses" of the cell and without them life would not exist. Mitochondrial dysfunction is shockingly common and lack of exercise, an unhealthy diet, aging, poor sleep, and chronic stress or disease can all damage the mitochondria.[102]

Mitochondrial dysfunction is associated with virtually every mental or neurological affliction on earth, including physiological stress, anxiety, depression, autism, cognitive deficits, Alzheimer's and Parkinson's disease, bipolar disorder, and schizophrenia .[103] It's also associated with chronic fatigue and an overactive immune system; and with increased inflammation and oxidative stress which are the two underlying causes of most chronic disease and pain conditions.[104] By helping to optimize mitochondrial functions, regular CVAC sessions can theoretically help reduce the risk for all of the above diseases and disorders.

Athletic and Fitness benefits

Spending time at a high altitude before training at a low altitude has been proven to result in a marked improvement in athletic performance.[105] The CVAC

[102]

[103] https://www.ncbi.nlm.nih.gov/pmc/articles/PMC5761714/
[104] https://www.ncbi.nlm.nih.gov/pmc/articles/PMC5761714/
[105]

https://www.businesswire.com/news/home/20060615005083/en/Researchers-University-Hawaii-Present-Scientific-Validation-Cyclic#.VOPbFBjB-IY machine simulates this and it accelerates the process by rapidly cycling between atmospheric pressures of varying altitudes. Because the exposure time is so short, it likely does so without impairing recovery.[106]

By challenging the body to adapt to changes in air pressure, improvements in mitochondrial function, red blood cell count, and oxygen saturation occur. This in turn, improves athletic performance, endurance, and recovery. CVAC sessions have been found to provide the benefits of traditional exercise only much quicker and without the joint stress, lactic acid buildup, and muscle tearing that is often associated with these activities. Anecdotal reports suggest the CVAC may also give you a competitive edge by enhancing focus, concentration and reaction time, and reducing stress.

Stress Management Benefits

Many people who use the CVAC process report a notable improvement in stress management. Although the exact mechanism of action is unknown, Allan hypothesizes that this is likely linked at least in part to mitochondrial enhancement. Researchers have found mitochondria control heart rate and increase it as a part of the fight or flight response.[107] And a study published

---

[106]

https://www.businesswire.com/news/home/20060615005083/en/Researchers-University-Hawaii-Present-Scientific-Validation-Cyclic#.VOPbFBjB-IY

[107] https://www.ncbi.nlm.nih.gov/pmc/articles/PMC4398998/

in *Frontiers in Neuroendocrinology* journal shows mitochondria are intimately linked to stress, providing both the energy and signals that enable and direct stress adaptation. [108]

"A dirty living environment may be perceived as a threat," explains Allen. "Perhaps the anxiety response is produced by the mitochondria to get people to physically move to stimulate the lymphatic and glymphatic system to clean out their living environment...The vacuum and pressure cycling of the CVAC Process likely cleans out the mitochondria's living environment like exercise does and thereby calms the mitochondria's sensing of the threat."

Considerations

I myself have experienced the amazing benefits of CVAC and you can watch my session on YouTube here: https://www.youtube.com/watch?v=vEav8H320Q4 &feature=youtu.

If you would like more information on CVAC and on clinics offering sessions near you: http://cvacsystems.com/site/

Supportive Research

---

[108]
https://www.sciencedirect.com/science/article/pii/S0091302218300062

Mitochondrial Nanotunnels:
www.ncbi.nlm.nih.gov/pubmed/28935166

Editorial: Mitochondrial Communication in Physiology, Disease and Aging:
https://www.ncbi.nlm.nih.gov/pmc/articles/PMC6470183/

Mitochondrial-nuclear communications:
https://www.ncbi.nlm.nih.gov/pubmed/17227225/

Our (Mother's) Mitochondria and Our Mind:
https://www.ncbi.nlm.nih.gov/pmc/articles/PMC5761714/

Non-coding RNAs: the dark side of nuclear-mitochondrial communication:
http://m.emboj.embopress.org/content/36/9/1123

Mitochondria Communication:
https://www.keystonesymposia.org/index.cfm?e=Web.Meeting.Flyer&MeetingID=1447

Support Your Gut Health

The bacteria in your gut send signals to the mitochondria and the signals they send have a direct impact on mitochondrial health, functioning and aging. Unfortunately, very few of us have healthy gut microbiomes because the beneficial bacteria are killed off by things such as the Standard American Diet, stress, antibiotics, certain medications, and chemicals in the water we drink. To repopulate your gut, eat fermented foods such as pickled vegetables, miso, and kombucha and take a high-quality probiotic with at least 25,000 billion live active bacteria per serving. We use the freshest source of probiotics mixed with Vitamin D3 to support gut health and the immune system.

Support Mitochondria with Nutrients

Certain herbs and nutrients help to protect mitochondria from oxidative damage and improve mitochondrial function, including: CoQ10[109], alpha lipoic acid[110], berberine[111], bergamot[112], and lycopene.[113]

Insulin Heart Stability contains the above mitochondria boosting nutrients, as well as probiotics to support gut health, vitamin D3 and

[109] https://pubmed.ncbi.nlm.nih.gov/11796022/
[110] https://pubmed.ncbi.nlm.nih.gov/17605107/
[111] https://www.sciencedirect.com/science/article/pii/S0925443911002316
[112] https://pubmed.ncbi.nlm.nih.gov/28758404/
[113] https://pubmed.ncbi.nlm.nih.gov/28758404/

several additional immune boosting herbs and nutrients. See appendix section 1 for more info and the complete ingredients list.

5 steps to enhance immunity

1. Gargle with warm salt water regularly
2. Drink warm water regularly
3. Take Testro Plus daily; it contains three different types of bioavailable zinc to boost immunity, as well as cordyceps, astragalus, cinnamon bark, ginseng and several other herbs that activate your body's natural defense system.
4. Get Testro Genin and apply it to your neck and chest area daily. It contains bioavailable zinc, DIM and DHEA to bolster your immune system:
5. Take infrared saunas regularly to heat your core temperature to stimulate your immune system.

Section 4:

What to Do
If You Get Sick

Chapter 13:

Ten Steps to Support and Hasten Recovery from Illness

There is a ton of information available now on how to prevent virus infections but very little information on what to do if you or a loved one contracts one. In this chapter, you will learn ten steps you can take to detoxify, nutrify and fortify, and hasten the recovery process.

If You Contract an Infectious Disease:

The most important thing you can do aside from resting and eating the right diet is to increase your hydration with clean purified water (the best filters are Echo device or "Living Water," and reverse osmosis). This is important because fever dehydrates you, and dehydration makes the mucus in your nose, throat, and lungs dry up, which in turn clogs sinuses and respiratory tubes. Plus, your body needs fluids to fight the infection and flush-out toxins, and staying hydrated helps keep the mucus running, which is one of our natural defenses.

1. The best liquids to consume while sick are fresh, filtered water, herbal teas, soups, and cold-pressed juices. Avoid alcohol, and caffeinated and sugar-containing beverages because they hamper immunity, hinder sleep, and dehydrate you. Monitor your urine - if you are properly hydrated it will be clear; if it is yellow or orange it's a sign you are severely dehydrated and need to consume more liquids.

2. Consume a whole-foods, plant-based diet to nutrify and increase hydration, and move away from animal protein, dairy, caffeine, and alcohol because they severely dehydrate you. *See the next chapter for specifics on what you should and shouldn't be eating.

3. To turbocharge your immunity, you should aim to consume at least 64 oz. of blended nutrient-rich juice daily. Emphasize high water content fruits such as watermelon, oranges, jackfruit, and pineapple. For the best results, juice your vegetables (the Omega juicer is recommended) and then add the vegetable juice plus whole fruits into a 500 to 1000 horsepower blender (e.g. Hamilton Beach blender, Vitamix, etc.). The best vegetables to juice while sick are raw yams

and beets because they contain tons of vitamin C. They also increase nitric oxide in the body, which is one of the most versatile players in the immune system and involved in the pathogenesis and control of infectious diseases.

4. Nutrify your body even further by adding Grow Muscle Burn Fat to your juices. The organic beets in this product increase nitric oxide. It also contains MSM, Vitamin C, and niacin to detoxify, and amino acids which help rebuild weak tissue. To further support immunity add Acerola powder to your juice as well; it is one of the richest and most bioavailable sources of vitamin C.

5. Eat whole apples because they are rich in CH3 methyl donors. Methyl donors are required for methylation, and as explored earlier in the book - methylation is a vital metabolic process that occurs in every single cell and organ of your body. It turns genes on and off, synthesizes important hormones, plays a vital role in detoxification, supports immunity, and fights infections. To ensure you are getting enough methyl donors for optimal methylation and healing, take either DNA Protector or Mental Focus daily (see appendix for more information on methylation).

6. If you have a sore throat, gargle several times a day with sea salt stirred into warm purified water.

7. Do Not break the "fever" with Acetaminophen (Tylenol) or Ibuprofen (Advil). The fever is an important immune system defense mechanism that helps your body fight off bugs. It's not a function you want to suppress unless it reaches dangerously high levels, in which case massive hydration provided by a nutritional IV can be lifesaving. An emergency medicine doctor who is highly trained in the risk versus benefit of bringing a fever down can make this type of decision. Anil Bajnath, MD, explains there are known conditions where the appropriate therapy must be administered. However, be very clear, Big Pharma has made a huge profit off people believing that fevers are bad, when in fact, the fever is part of your body's amazing defense system.

8. Do Not take conventional cough medicines such as Mucinex, Robitussin and DayQuil/NyQuil. They are loaded with sugar, alcohol and chemicals which will weaken your immune system and slow down recovery. Another reason not to take these medicines is that similar to the fever,

coughing is an important part of the immune system's defense mechanism, and you want to support it, not suppress it.

9. Take hydrocortisone prescribed by an anti-aging doctor. This will typically reverse the disease within a day or two. To resolve dry cough, sore throat, and malaise use hydrocortisone cream (available by cream as 1% over the counter) - and take 20 mg cortisol tablets, 4 times a day for 48 hours. Once resolved, take 10 mg 4 x a day (please do so under the supervision of your healthcare provider).

10. Take the Immunity Fortification 6-pack to hasten recovery.

Chapter 14:

Why You Need to Feed a Fever and What to Feed It

"Feed a cold, starve a fever" is an adage that has been traced all the way back to a 1574 dictionary. But just because it's been a common adage for centuries doesn't mean it's correct. In fact, there are volumes of research including a *Scientific American* study covering nearly 100 years of research that shows you should feed a cold *and* feed a fever. In this chapter, you'll learn why it's so important to eat when you are sick and receive dietary guidelines for recovering from all types of infectious diseases.

Why You Need to Feed a Fever

The reasoning behind the adage: "Feed a cold, starve a fever" was that eating food helps the body generate warmth, which is needed during a cold. With the flu, however, there is a fever and heat already happening in the body, so avoiding food was thought to be helpful as a way to avoid "overheating." This is faulty logic though because the fever is an important immune system defense mechanism that helps the body fight off bugs; it's not a function you want to suppress unless it reaches dangerously high levels, in which case massive hydration provided by a nutritional IV can be life-saving.

You also need nutrients and energy to fight off infections and starving yourself deprives your body of both. In fact, the greater the fever, the more important it is that you eat because your energy demands increase with every degree your temperature rises. Another reason eating is essential when you have a fever is that if you don't, triglycerides from your body fat may be released. This is problematic because higher fat levels in the blood will make your insulin inefficient and hinder its ability to push energy into the cells for a stronger immune system.

White Blood Cell Efficiency SUPERCHARGERS!

And why you should eat them!

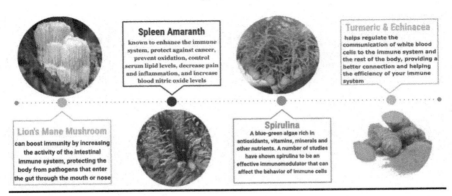

Spleen Amaranth
known to enhance the immune system, protect against cancer, prevent oxidation, control serum lipid levels, decrease pain and inflammation, and increase blood nitric oxide levels

Turmeric & Echinacea
helps regulate the communication of white blood cells to the immune system and the rest of the body, providing a better connection and helping the efficiency of your immune system

Lion's Mane Mushroom
can boost immunity by increasing the activity of the intestinal immune system, protecting the body from pathogens that enter the gut through the mouth or nose

Spirulina
A blue-green algae rich in antioxidants, vitamins, minerals and other nutrients. A number of studies have shown spirulina to be an effective immunomodulator that can affect the behavior of immune cells

The Best Diet for Cold, and Flu

While recovering from an illness, the two most important things you can do are to get enough rest and to eat properly. That does not mean overeat; that means eat within a window of 8 a.m. to 8 p.m. If you eat late at night, be sure to eat light foods such as fruit, vegetables and/or tubers prepared without oil.

Although fasting while sick is not advised, there are certain foods that you should avoid. For starters, you should eliminate all animal products because they increase inflammation and dehydrate you. Meat and dairy are also loaded with disease-causing microbes (salmonella, e. Coli, viral load, etc.), as well as antibiotics that diminish your healthy bacteria, and toxins that suppress your immune system. You should also cut out sugar, processed foods, and all oils and foods that contain oil -- these foods are void of nutrients, they increase inflammation, and they suppress your immune system.

We must have sufficient glucose from whole plant-based foods to fuel the red blood cells, white blood cells, and maintain higher oxygen levels. Eat more easy-to-digest plant foods that are rich in antioxidants, nitrates (beets), and water content. Make sure to include a lot of fruit -- the more you consume, the more hydrated you will be, and hydration supports the fever in doing its job of killing off harmful microbes.

Ideally, you should choose vegetable-based soups over chicken soup. There is nothing particularly healthy about chicken soup; it's only beneficial because it provides energy and hydration and the warm vapor moistens dried mucus. Vegetable soup will provide the same benefits plus additional nutrients.

Citrus and fresh chilis are particularly beneficial, as they are concentrated sources of vitamin C, and chilis have the added benefit of improving blood flow, stimulating mucus membranes, and fighting infections. Make sure you get plenty of fiber as well, as this will help stimulate the colon and the release of toxins.

Considerations

Most people lose their appetites when their bodies are fighting an infection. If you are finding it difficult to eat, then consume fresh cold press vegetable juices without any additives; they help supply essential nutrients and energy in condensed form. You can also take a scoop of Slim Blend Pro powder combined with Grow Muscle Burn Fat in the morning, afternoon, and evening. Also, I find fresh fruit is best eaten rather raw than juiced when working to recover from fever or infectious disease.

Chapter 15:

Breakthrough All-Natural Therapies!

What We Now Know

Frontline researchers have discovered some pathogens cause hemolysis, which is the destruction of red blood cells (RBCs) and prolonged and progressive hypoxia (starving your body of oxygen). They do this by binding to the heme groups in hemoglobin in the red blood cells and causing the hemoglobin to lose its iron ion, which in turn strips its ability to carry oxygen throughout the body. Those freed iron ions are then able to roam throughout the body, leading to elevated ferritin levels, and this combination of high ferritin and low oxygen leads to oxidative damage and inflammation, and all that nasty stuff you see in CT scans of a patient's lungs.[114]

These new insights mean the strokes and the organ failures leading to death are not caused by any traditional form of Acute Respiratory Distress Syndrome (ARDS) or pneumonia, which is the

---

[114] https://journals.physiology.org/doi/pdf/10.1152/ajplung.00312.2016

assumption doctors have been operating on. They are happening because people are desaturating (losing oxygen in their blood) and because the free iron is causing systemic damage, alveolar inflammation, and coagulation.[115] [116]

Hyperbaric oxygen therapy (HBOT), which has been used for over 75 years, may offer us the safest and most effective solution, especially when used in conjunction with lifestyle medicine protocols which we will explore in more depth at my blog and podcasts.

Vitamin C - Nature's Safe and All-Natural Solution

Vitamin C is well known as an immune system booster, and it supports lymphocytes, neutrophils, and other important regulators of the immune system, but it's effects on pathogenic diseases goes beyond just supporting immunity. L-ascorbic acid (the natural form of vitamin C which can come from supplements derived from fruits, kiwi, chili spice, peppers) supports all cellular redox reactions, immune responses, and mitochondria; and perhaps most importantly it can help prevent hypoxia and lower cell-free hemoglobin.[117] The reason why some patients are

---

[115] https://www.ncbi.nlm.nih.gov/pmc/articles/PMC4772369/
[116] https://journals.physiology.org/doi/pdf/10.1152/ajplung.00312.2016
[117] https://www.ncbi.nlm.nih.gov/pmc/articles/PMC4772369/

difficult to oxygenate is that there is a systematic destruction of red blood cells, resulting in cell-free heme that has oxidized iron ions in the ferric state, and ascorbic acid helps prevent this from happening.

Foods To Avoid to Improve White Blood Cell Quantity

Toxic heated or excessively processed foods harm the immune system

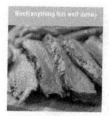 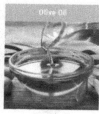

Meat(Anything but well done)	Soda	Chocolate	Olive Oil
What lowers the number of white blood cells available to fight pathogens more than more pathogens? Meat not cooked thoroughly is our number one source of pathogen exposure in the modern food chain	Extremely high in calories and low in everything but synthetic chemicals. There is no more surefire a way to hit a calorie surplus and nutrient deficit simultaneously than to have sodas and sugary beverages as a staple part of your daily or weekly routines	Cocoa in its raw and unprocessed form isn't the problem. But when you add dairy and sugar it all of a the sudden becomes a immune system and Hormonal nightmare	Touted as a health food by the uninformed. Olive oil just like any other oil processed out of its natural form is mechanically debilitating to our immune system

Now for good news: A new study has found high doses of oral Vitamin C (10 grams) is absorbed into the bloodstream as effectively as IVC is. [118] It was previously believed that the body could only absorb a small amount of oral vitamin C at a time, but this new research may prove that assumption wrong. Here is what the Townsend Letter (we await peer review journals to confirm or deny the effectiveness of Vitamin

---

[118] Owen Fonorow and Steve Hickey 2020 Unexpected Early Response in Oral Bioavailability of Ascorbic Acid – Townsend Letter March 13, 2020, prior to print publication.
https://www.townsendletter.com/article/online-unexpected-oral-vitamin-c-response/

C while my personal research has indicated hyperbaric oxygen therapy can improve the therapy outcome), who reported this study advice for patients:

The following supplementation guide for oral ascorbic acid is offered for informational purposes only and should *NOT be considered as MEDICAL ADVICE.*

- *Initial onset of symptoms:*
- *3 to 5 g in one dose, followed by 1 g every 30 to 60 mins for the following 3 hours. Repeat this cycle until symptoms subside.*
- *Milder cases:*
- *2 to 5 g in one dose, followed by 1 g every hour for the following 4 – 6 hours. Repeat this cycle until symptoms subside.*
- *Severe/critical cases:*
- *10 g in one dose, followed by 2 g every 15 to 30 mins for the following 2 hours. Repeat this cycle until symptoms improve."*

As a rule, the higher gram dosages are best used for emergency use. For prevention, 200 mg from natural sources such as Tart Cherry, Rose Hips, and Acerola Cherry may be best. These natural sources are incredibly high in bioflavonoids which are polyphenolic compounds found in plants; they are also more bioavailable and better absorbed than synthetic vitamin C. Tart cherry can be found in a product called Stay Young Chewable, and a powder product called Grow Muscle Burn Fat.

During flu season, consume plenty of oranges, bell peppers, and chili peppers - they are even higher in natural bioavailable Vitamin C than synthetic man-made Vitamin C supplements. The countries that consume the most chili peppers have the lowest incidence of colds and flu. This is not only because of the vitamin C content but the capsicum in peppers stimulates the lungs to clear toxins and clear phlegm from the lungs and throat. Also worth noting the white part just under the orange or tangerine peel are the richest source of vitamin C and bioflavonoids.

Vitamin and Intravenous Therapy (IV)

Dr. David Brownstein has had a high degree of success with over 100 of his sick patients using a holistic protocol that includes oral dosing of vitamins A, C, D, and iodine as well as IV vitamin C, ozone, and hydrogen peroxide.[119] Dr. Brownstein has been using this combination of vitamins to support the immune system and treat viral infections successfully for years. "I (and my partners) have no doubt that the vast majority of patients would avoid a deterioration of their symptoms if they started this protocol at the onset of symptoms," states Brownstein.

---

[119] https://www.drbrownstein.com/virus-xiv:-the-good-news-is-still-there-but-not-reported-by-msm/

Cortisone

Many leading experts in bioidentical hormone therapy believe Hydrocortisone (trade name Cortef, also available in generic form, https://www.drugs.com/availability/generic-cortef.html) can be used. This would be the least costly option and could lead to a chance of rapid recovery. This adrenal support therapy using natural cortisol was discovered to be incredibly effective to reverse or stabilize most symptoms (dry cough, malaise, fever).

The following guide for cortisone by Dr. William Jefferies in his book "Safe Uses of Cortisol," is offered for informational purposes only, and should NOT be considered as MEDICAL ADVICE. Please consult with your healthcare provider before taking cortisone.

"Take the following dosages of natural cortisol about three to four hours apart: 20 mg upon waking, 20 mg noon, 20 mg afternoon, and 20 mg evening, which is to be "taken until the patient feels well" which typically occurs within three to four days. Then reduce by half dosage to 10 mg four times a day divided equally for two days. Then 5 mg four times daily for two days, then stop.

"This protocol will be most effective for those with pre-existing problems like chronic fatigue, and it has even been shown effective in those stricken with serious deadly pathogens. This approach saved hundreds of lives as reported by William McKinnley

Jefferies based upon preliminary treatment outcome reports during the years 2018 to 2020. When this therapy was first used in influenza patients, antibiotics (erythromycin or penicillin) were used for seven days, yet all subsequent patients have received cortisol without antibiotics.

"I achieved great success using the following advanced immune rejuvenation approach: sun exposure, cold press juices, hormone optimization, and Adrenal Immune Support (4 am, 4 noon, 4 pm, 4 evening). Along with Cortef (start at 20 mg, then 10 mg then 5 mg as outlined above), and hydrocortisone cream 1% (from Mexico 2%) applied to the skin daily for optimal levels of cortisone. Suzie Shuder, MD, has written a paper on this therapy related to Hypercortisolemia which every doctor and healthcare professional should read and consider offering for immune disorder, severe drug addictions, food addiction, over eating, and those who thrive on drama (needing an emotional high to get a quick release of cortisol to feel good again)."

Chapter 16:

Stem Cells for Prevention, and for Recovery in the Terminally Ill

There is a novel therapy that almost no one is talking about that can protect you from serious illnesses and be used for rapid recovery.

What It Is

The novel therapy that can protect and heal us is stem cell therapy. Stem cells are the primary repair system of the body, and they divide essentially without limit to replenish other cells. When they divide, they either become new cells or specialized cells with a specific function. Stem cells decline with age, and it is this decline that is responsible for most of the symptoms and diseases associated with aging, as well as the body's reduced ability to repair itself.[120][121]

How Stem Cells Affect Your Immune System

Stem cells are required for the production of vital immune system cells that are crucial for fighting infections and other diseases.[122] In fact, stem cells produce approximately 10 billion new white blood cells (immune cells including T cells, B cells and NK cells) every single day.[123] Several types of stem cells also act to suppress the activities of infective viruses and viral DNA.

Mesenchymal Stem Cells (MSCs)

Mesenchymal stem cells (MSCs) are considered particularly beneficial for the immune system. Studies have found MSCs have several properties that may make them very useful for infections, including:[124]

- Potent anti-inflammatory and immune regulatory functions
- A unique ability to travel to damaged tissues

---

[120] https://www.ncbi.nlm.nih.gov/pmc/articles/PMC5316899/
[121] https://hsci.harvard.edu/aging-0
[122] https://www.sciencedaily.com/releases/2020/03/200313112148.htm
[123] https://www.sciencedaily.com/releases/2018/05/180530113147.htm
[124] https://www.ncbi.nlm.nih.gov/pmc/articles/PMC6022321/

- The ability to regenerate and repair damaged tissues and reduce tissue damage

Stem Cells for Healing

Preliminary research on mice has found MSCs are able to reduce pathogen-induced lung injury and mortality. In these studies, MSCs were found to reduce inflammation and the number of inflammatory cells that enter the lungs after contracting a disease such as pneumonia. Researchers believe stem cells can be used to repair damaged tissues in the respiratory system and promote faster healing and recovery, and they are conducting studies to prove this theory. [125]

How to Boost Stem Cells

Maintaining healthy stem cell levels will support your immune system so it can fight off disease. Although beneficial for everyone, it is especially important to boost your stem cells if you are elderly or sick. Stem cell therapy injections can rapidly replenish your stem cell supply, however, many types are illegal in the USA, and the legal ones are a major investment in your health, so much so that I personally have undergone multiple types of stem cell therapies (I

---

[125] https://www.scmp.com/news/china/society/article/3052495/virus-far-more-likely-sars-bond-human-cells-scientists-say

choose not to do embryonic stem cells, nor will I do fat derived stem cells) including advancements with Very Small Embryonic-Like Stem Cells (VSELs) as reported in the medical journal *Circulation* that are dormant stem cells that have remained ageless within our own bodies.
https://www.ahajournals.org/doi/10.1161/CIRCRES AHA.118.314287

Fight Disease and Aging with Stem Cell Enhancer:
*Stem Cell Enhancer is a complete body rejuvenation formula with superfoods and herbs to boost stem cell production, optimize immunity, reduce inflammation, support healthy joints, heal damaged tissue, address autoimmune disorders and help your body regenerate from any issue. By improving the release rate by 60% and colony count, you get a huge infusion of stem cells offered in no other product. In fact, studies showed a whopping 140% increase in stem cell colony counts inside the bone marrow after just six weeks of use! *See the appendix for the complete list of ingredients and benefits.*

Fortunately, you can boost stem cell count naturally by exercising regularly and consuming a whole-foods, plant-based diet that is high in fiber, fresh fruits and vegetables, herbs, and spices. Also, avoid sugar, animal products, and cigarettes; limit stress, optimize sleep, and make sure you get enough vitamin D, either through supplementation or by 15 minutes of daily sunlight exposure. For a more dramatic effect boost in stem cell production, take Stem Cell Enhancer.

Closing Thoughts

To help people build a healthy immune system, I think we should add substantial taxes to harmful substances such as alcohol, cigarettes, weed, opiates, animal protein products, and dairy. And the government should start allocating money towards wellness care.

Wellness Care Proposal

We should reward and provide tax incentives to people who take care of themselves as indicated by sobriety tests, exercise performance tests, and sleep logs. Fruits and vegetables should be subsidized so that a whole-foods, plant-based diet is affordable and accessible to all. To give the sick the best chance of recovery, whole food plant-based meals should be served in all hospitals, starting immediately. And the government should educate the public on the negative health impacts of sugar, animal products, and the excess use of vegetable or olive oil in your recipes. Acts of kindness should be awarded, and the importance of love and connection should be emphasized.

There are no signs of the sickcare paradigm being transformed into wellness care any time soon, so the onus is on us as individuals. American's need to educate themselves and make the lifestyle changes that are necessary for optimal health. That way when this is all over, we will be more immune to all types of infectious diseases. We will also dramatically lower our risk for chronic diseases such as diabetes and cancer, reduce our reliance on toxic prescription drugs, and become a happier, healthier, and longer-living society.

My Pledge to You

I promise to educate the people of the world "till the day I live" (not die) to see a time when all-natural methods of health and healing are understood, appreciated, and accepted as the front-line of defense to support our bodies' innate ability to recover from all illnesses and disease. An optimally functioning immune system is the safest way to protect ourselves and it is far more powerful than any Big Pharma solution.

Stay Healthy,
Nick Delgado

APPENDIX

1. Nutraceuticals for Immunity, Anti-Aging, and Optimum Health

The Delgado Protocol team of experts have spent decades researching, sourcing, formulating and optimizing clinically proven nutraceutical supplements that effectively address the most common underlying causes of aging, sickness and disease. We work alongside cutting-edge doctors to develop advanced clinical supplements, by doctors for doctors, and also for those who want certified, safe, and effective products. All these products are available at www.DocNutrients.com.

Our products are derived from the highest quality ingredients and contain no soy, no gluten, no dairy, no sugar, no GMOs, no stearates, no phosphates, no synthetic derivatives, and no harmful additives. They are made using Good Manufacturing Practices (GMP), at a certified laboratory in the USA that adheres to the highest standards. We are so confident in our products that we provide a 100% satisfaction money back guarantee. You have nothing to lose and exceptional health to gain!

Doc Nutrients - Quick Referral Guide

Immunity Fortification Pack

Adrenal Immune Support
DNA Protector
Insulin Heart Stability
Liver Accel
Stay Young Chewable
Stem Cell Enhancer

Additional Nutraceuticals for Health, Intimacy, Fitness, and Longevity

Clear Skin Advance
DHT Hair and Skin
Energy Extreme Complex
Grow Muscle Burn Fat
Mental Focus
Slim Blend Pro
Stay Lean
Stem Cell Strong
Testro Genin Cream
Testrogenesis
Testro Plus
Thyrodine

Immunity Fortification Pack

The immune fortification pack nutrients work synergistically with each other, helping to optimize all of the body's repair and defense systems, leading to a turbocharged immune system. For a special deal on these immune-boosting supplements with proprietary blended formulations designed by doctors, go to http://docnutrients.com/secret. For a limited time, everyone who purchases this Immunity Fortification Pack will also gain FREE access to the course Building a Strong Immunity.

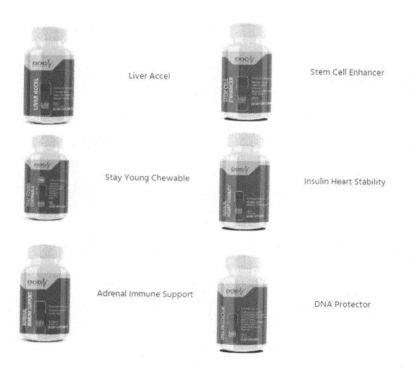

Liver Accel

Stem Cell Enhancer

Stay Young Chewable

Insulin Heart Stability

Adrenal Immune Support

DNA Protector

1. Adrenal Immune Support

Adrenal Immune Support is a clinically formulated nutraceutical that contains adrenal cortex and several adrenal optimizing, immune boosting, and energy enhancing herbs. It also contains herbs that help target RNA and DNA viruses. This proprietary combination helps your body manage stress (a major immune system destroyer), provides naturally occurring cortisol, and leads to an immediate boost in adrenal function and immunity. It also helps reduce addiction intensity and overeating, supports sleep, and helps toxins exit the liver.

This proprietary formula helped me reverse adrenal fatigue bordering on Addison disease. I have been taking it for over 10 years now, and if I miss a day, I still function well as my adrenal function has been restored. I have had multiple 24-hour urine tests, saliva tests taken morning, noon, afternoon, and evening, and have found in most cases my natural adrenal function works incredibly well even under massive levels of stress.

Dosage Guide for Prevention and Recovery

To support immune defenses, take three capsules morning and afternoon. If the cold, flu, or virus develops, increase your intake to 3-4 capsules, up to 4 times a day to ward off symptoms. My patients and the patients of many doctors we work with report great success and full recovery from serious cases of both arthritis and the flu following this protocol. While this supplement is recommended for anyone who wants to boost energy and gain added protection from infectious diseases, if you are on anabolic testosterone boosters, you are elderly, sick, or have a chronic disease, this immunity booster becomes even more critical.

Adrenal Immune Support

Benefits of Doc Nutrients Adrenal Immune Support ™

- Healthy Stress Management
- Better Mood and Sleep Quality
- Improved Biochemistry
- Increased Energy
- Immune Support

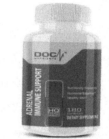

Proprietary Adrenal Cortex Blend: Dimethylglycine HCL, Cranberry Extract, Grapefruit Seed Extract, Garlic Bulb Extract, Caprylic Acid (as Sodium Caprylate), Tea Tree Leaf Powder, Sensoril™ Ashwagandha (Withania Somnifera) Root and Leaf Extract, Licorice Root Powder, Adrenal Cortex, Policosanol, Echinacea Purpurea Herb Extract, Wild Cherry Bark Powder, Lomatium Root Powder.

Adrenal Immune Support
Potent enhancer of immune system, reduces stress, addictions, and overeating.
Helps toxins exit the liver and supports sleep!

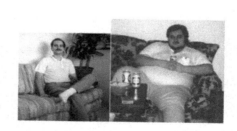
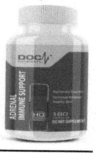

2. DNA Protector

DNA Protector is a powerful methylation boosting product, formulated by leading anti-aging experts. It contains all of the key methyl donor nutrients outlined above as well as several B-vitamins which also act as methyl donors, dramatically improving methylation.[126] It helps your body in its one billion chemical reactions per second, and as it does so, the CH3 molecule helps to prevent the breakdown of the cells and restore energy reserves.

The special ingredient combination in DNA Protector helps to process toxic chemicals that you are exposed to on a daily basis and reduces the toxic build-up and inflammation that leads to weakened immunity. It also supports the suppression of viral DNA, re-energizes your body, helps you reach peak performance, protects you from damaging phone towers, slows the signs of aging, increases your mental performance, boosts energy and athletic recovery, clears bad estrogens, combats depression, and regulates mood. Unlike cheaper products, the B vitamins in this formula are provided in their most bioavailable form, which makes them far more effective at supporting methylation.

126

https://www.researchgate.net/publication/11222486_Diet_Methyl_Don ors_and_DNA_Methylation_Interactions_between_Dietary_Folate_Met hionine_and_Choline

- 5G
- Viruses
- Autism Spectrum
- Athletic Recovery
- Cognitive Support
- Clears Bad Estrogens

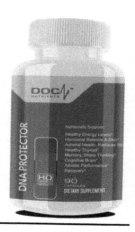

3. Insulin Heart Stability

To boost mitochondria and increase oxygen transport by reducing lipids, use <u>Insulin Heart Stability</u>. This supplement also helps to reduce cholesterol, improve the immune system, boost cardiovascular health, stabilizes insulin and metabolic syndrome, supports healthy brain function and prostate health, and helps with ovarian cysts and healthier skin. It contains vitamin D3 and zinc in their most bioavailable forms, as well as licorice root, cinnamon, chromium, and Amla. It also contains several additional immune-supporting nutrients including olive leaf powder, probiotics, bergamot orange fruit extract, and alpha-lipoic acid.

Insulin Heart Stability™

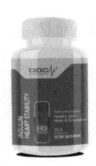

- Immune System Enhancer
- Improves Cardiovascular Health, Manages LDL Cholesterol
- Stabilizes Insulin & Metabolic Syndrome
- Supports Healthy Brain Function
- Helps with Ovarian Cysts & PCOS (Polycystic Ovarian Syndrome)
- Supports Prostate Health

Proprietary Blend: *Lactobacillus Acidophilus Complex, Maca Root Powder, Chaste Tree Fruit Powder, Berberine HCl, Garcinia Fruit Extract, Rasberry Leaf Powder, Chinese Peony Root Powder, Gymnema Leaf Powder, Chia Seed Powder, ConcenTrace Trace Mineral Powder, Prickly Pear Leaf Cactus Powder, Pumpkin Seed Powder, Olive Leaf Powder, Amla (Embilca officinalis) Fruit Powder, Artichoke Leaf Powder, Organic Cassia Bark Powder, Licorice Root Powder, Policosonol, Alpha Lipoic Acid, Co Enzyme Q10, Lycopene* **Other Ingredients:** *Hypromellose (capsule), Rice Flour* **Active Ingredients:** *Vitamin D (as Cholecalciferol) 125mcg, Zinc (as Zinc Gluconate and Zinc Sulfate) 3mg, Chromium (as Chromium Polynicotinate) 200mcg, Bergamonte (Bergamot Orange Fruit Extract) 500mg*

4. Liver Accel

If you want to support your liver so it can properly eliminate toxins and excess hormones, reduce inflammation and mount a strong immune response, start taking Liver Accel daily. This clinically formulated supplement contains milk thistle which helps your liver regenerate new, healthy cells. It also contains astragalus root which helps fight stress (a major immune system saboteur), and a blend of antioxidant dense super herbs that support liver function, fight inflammation, reduce oxidative damage, and bolster the immune system. D-Tox helps prevent and reverse estrogen dominance, the negative symptoms associated with testosterone therapy, and with time, it also helps support healthy immunity.

Liver Accel

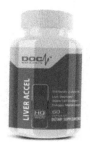

Benefits of Liver Accel™

- Helps detoxify hormones from fat cells
- Can be used as part of an acne protocol
- Can be used as part of an Estrogen Dominance related weight loss protocol
- Can be used with bio identical hormone therapies
- Can be used as part of a cancer immune support protocol

Proprietary Blend: *Astragalus Root Extract, Turmeric Root Powder, Cyperus Root Powder, Asparagus Shoot Powder, Sunflower Lecithin Powder, Pomegranate Fruit Extract, Ginger Root Powder, Silymarin (from Milk Thistle Seed Extract), Wasabi Root Powder.* **Other Ingredients:** *Hypromellose (capsule), Rice Flour.* **Active Ingredients:** *Vitamin E 24mg (as d-alpha tocopheryl succinate).*

5. Stay Young Chewable

Stay Young chewable is a great supplement to take daily for enhancing your love life, slowing the aging process, and supporting the immune system. It contains alpha lipoic acid, Coenzyme Q-10, DNA, RNA and phosphatidylcholine to support the repair of malaria-like misshapen cells and telomeres, and helps to boost health, immunity, and vitality.

It also contains nutrients that boost nitric oxide (master neurotransmitter) production, which is one of the most versatile players in the immune system and involved in the pathogenesis and control of infectious diseases. Nitric oxide enhances libido, stamina and pleasure, and sleep quality. Many of my clients report a noticeable increase in libido and pleasure sensations immediately after starting this supplement, and women report an increase in lubrication and orgasmic intensity while taking it.

Stay Young Chewable

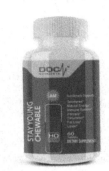

Benefits of Stay Young Chewable (AM formula) Tablets

- Telomere Support
- Nitric Oxide (master neurotransmitter) production
- Intimacy Support
- Sleep support
- Free of Soy, Dairy, Artificial Coloring, Gluten, and Preservatives; Easily Chewable, tasty

Proprietary Blend: Spleen Amaranth (Red Spinach) Leaf Powder, Beet Root Extract, L-Citrulline, Collards (Kale) Leaf Powder, Pomegranate Fruit Powder, Astragalus Root Extract, Spinach Leaf Powder, Betaine HCl, Hawthorn Berry Extract, Stevia Leaf Extract, L-Carnosine, Acetyl-L-Carnitine HCl, Alpha Lipoic Acid, CoEnzyme Q10, DNA (Deoxyribonucleic Acid), RNA (Ribonucleic Acid). **Other Ingredients:** Xylitol, Natural Flavors, Silicon Dioxide.

6. Stem Cell Enhancer

Stem Cell Enhancer is a complete body rejuvenation formula with superfoods and herbs to boost stem cell production, optimize immunity, reduce inflammation, support healthy joints, heal damaged tissue, address autoimmune disorders and help your body regenerate from any issue. By improving the release rate by 60% and colony count, you get a huge infusion of stem cells offered in no other product. In fact, studies showed a whopping 140% increase in stem cell colony counts inside the bone marrow after just six weeks of use!

The proprietary blend of nutrients in Stem Cell Enhancer also helps to reduce binding proteins and to stimulate natural growth hormone production, so the stem cells get the best environment to begin their healing work. It contains deer antler (this may confer an unfair advantage to athletes, so check with regulating bodies to verify your sport allows this supplement) and helps restore hemoglobin to red blood cells. It also contains medicinal mushrooms which rapidly repair damage in the lungs and body. Plus, it provides antioxidants to ward off aging caused by free radicals as well as several immune-boosting, energy-increasing, and anti-inflammatory nutrients.

See my website videos and blogs for the incredible benefits of stem cells for antiaging recovery.

Stem Cell Enhancer

Benefits of Stem Cell Enhancer™

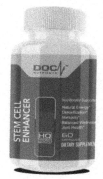

- Natural Energy
- Detoxification
- Immunity
- Balanced Wellness
- Joint Health
- Addresses Autoimmune Disorders

Proprietary Blend: *Velvet Deer Antler, Spirulina Plant Powder, Cordyceps Plant Mushroom, Maitake Mushroom Powder, Reishi Mushroom Powder, Lion's Mane Mushroom Powder, Tremella Mushroom Powder, Agaricus Mushroom Powder, Japanese Knotweed Root Powder, Cabbage Palm Berry Extract, Blueberry Fruit Extract, Brown Seaweed Extract.*
Other Ingredients: *Gelatin (Capsule), Microcrystalline Cellulose.*

Additional Nutraceuticals for Health, Intimacy, Fitness, and Longevity

7. Clear Skin Advance

Clear Skin Advance

Clear Skin Advance TM (regular strength) is designed to support the clearing of toxic estrogens, while supporting the production of healthy estrogens. Both men and women are profoundly affected by estrogens. Some are natural, and some are what we call xenoestrogens which originate outside the body. The use of things like, plastics, pesticides, chemicals, bad fats and oils, processed foods, preservatives, and pollution, to name a few, have dramatically altered our biochemistry. Most acne is caused by toxic estrogen buildup. These synthetic estrogens also contribute to cancers.

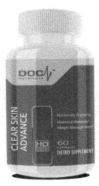

Benefits of Clear Skin AdvanceTM

- Can be used as part of an acne protocol
- Helps detoxify harmful types of estrogen hormones from fat cells
- Can be used as part of an Estrogen Dominance related weight loss protocol
- Can be used with bioidentical hormone therapies

Proprietary DIM Complex: *DIM (Diindolylmethane), Indole-3-Carbinol, Sunflower Lecithin Powder.* **Other Ingredients:** *Hypromellose (capsule), Rice Flour.* **Active Ingredients:** *13.4mg Vitamin E (as d-aplha tocopheryl succinate).*

Nature has provided us with a potent natural solution for people who have high androgens, estrogens, or prolactin levels and are experiencing acne, man boobs, or compromised immunity as a result. This solution is called diindolylmethane, or DIM and it is found naturally in cruciferous vegetables. DIM increases the production of SHBG, detoxifies harmful chemicals, shifts bad estrogens into healthy estrogens, and reduces excess hormones. In order to get clinically effective doses of DIM, take the internationally acclaimed nutraceutical Clear Skin Advance - each serving provides doses of DIM that are equivalent to consuming 10 pounds of cruciferous vegetables.

8. DHT Hair and Skin

DHT Hair and Skin contains DIM, which helps clear out excess estrogens from the body, which if left untreated can impair immune function and lead to autoimmunity. This nutraceutical also contains beta-sitosterol, which gives it the ability to calm down Dihydro-testosterone (DHT) and androgen activity. Take DHT Hair and Skin instead of EstroBlock if you have acne plus any of the following signs of too much DHT: loss of scalp hair at the temples and on the crown, increased body and facial hair, excess sweating, and aggressive feelings or episodes.

DHT Hair & Skin

DHT Hair & Skin is the perfect complement to our Hormone Cleans Pro for men or Clean Skin Advanced for women. DHT Hair & Skin has beta-sitosterols, which gives it the ability to calm down Dihydrotestosterone (DHT) and androgen activity in the skin! The cruciferous mix of natural vegetable extracts in DHT Hair & Skin provides a unique concentration of isothiocyanates and glucosinolates offering your body protection by neutralizing potentially harmful estrogen metabolites (16aOHE) and xenoestrogens (estrogen-like environmental chemicals). This boosts cell protection.

Proprietary Blend: *Cabbage Leaf Powder, Astragalus Root Powder, Turmeric Root Powder, DIM (Diindolylmethane), Parsley Leaf Extract, Broccoli Sprout Extract, Celery Seed Extract, Rosemary Leaf Extract, Pomegranate Fruit Powder, Sesame Seed Powder, beta-Sitosterol (from Pine Bark Extract).* **Other Ingredients:** *Hypromellose (capsule), Rice Flour.* **Active Ingredients:** *Vitamin E 18 IU (as d-alpha tocopheryl succinate).*

9. Energy Extreme Complex

Energy Extreme Complex

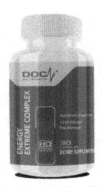

Benefits of Energy Extreme ComplexTM

- Supports Improved Athletic Performance
- Supports Improved Metabolism
- Supports Healthy Telomeres
- Enhances Mental Concentration & Focus

Proprietary Blend: Guarana Seed Extract, Caffeine Anhydrous, Kudzu Root Powder, Green Tea Leaf Extract, Cordyceps Fruiting Body Extract, American Ginseng Root Extract, DNA, RNA **Other Ingredients**: Hypromellose (capsule), Rice Flour.

Suggested use: Take 1 capsule 30 minutes prior to activity. Be sure to hydrate with extra water. Consult with your health professional if you are taking medication. This formulation contains caffeine.

10. Grow Muscle Burn Fat

You can eat the healthiest diet in the world and still get sick if your body is toxic, or you are not properly absorbing the nutrients you are consuming (which most of us aren't). If you're serious about protecting yourself, start consuming Grow Muscle Burn Fat. This potent nutraceutical contains several bioavailable nutrients that get rapidly absorbed and utilized by your body and support your immune system in doing its job.

This formula also contains concentrated beetroot which releases a molecule called nitric oxide that plays a vital role in immunity and is involved in the pathogenesis and control of infectious diseases. Nitric oxide also helps oxygenate your blood and enhances the flow of nutrients throughout your body. Beets are also rich in immune boosting-phytochemicals and one serving of Grow Muscle Burn Fat provides 500% of your daily value of vitamin C.

The growth hormone complex is combined with amino acids that release HGH and other healing growth factors. It also contains MSM, niacin, and l-arginine -- all three of which help the body detoxify and repair lungs. L-arginine has the added benefit of helping the liver regenerate new and healthy cells. Plus it contains a blend of bioavailable amino acids and protein peptides that support healthy cells, promote fat burning and lean body mass, aid in gut health, reduce workout recovery time, enhance sleep and reduce inflammation -- all of which support healthy immune defenses. And as an added bonus, it is delicious!

Grow Muscle Burn Fat™

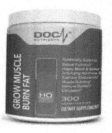

Highlights:

- *Organic, concentrated Beetroot for maximum nitric oxide production*
- *Formulated with bioavailable ingredients, for increased absorption and effectiveness*
- *Contains niacin and l-arginine for enhanced nitric oxide synthesis*
- *GMP certified*
- *Non-GMO*
- *Yeast, dairy, gluten, soy and preservative-free*
- *Delicious*

Exclusive anti-aging formula with bioavailable protein peptides (vegan) and nitric oxide, to help you look and feel years younger. Experience explosive energy, dramatically improved sports performance and stamina, quicker recovery time, rejuvenating sleep, and renewed cellular and organ health!

11. Mental Focus

Mental Focus™

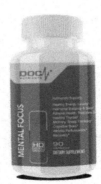

Mental Focus

- **Helps regulate Mood**
- **Helps manage PMS**
- **Helps address Fibroids**
- **Helps address depression**
- **Helps address endometriosis**
- **Helps support healthy brain function**

Proprietary Blend: Thiamine, Riboflavin, Vitamin B6, Folic Acid, Vitamin B12 (as Methylcobalamin), Biotin, Pantothenic Acid, Methylsulfonylmethane, Betaine Anhydrous, Dimethylglycine HCL, PhosphatidylSerine

12. Slim Blend Pro

Supplement Facts

Serving Size 2 scoops (about 19g)
Servings Per Container 20

	Amount per serving	% Daily Value
Calories	60	
Total Fat	1 g	1%*
Total Carbohydrate	6 g	2%*
Dietary Fiber	5 g	18%
Protein	10 g	
Vitamin C	1 mg	1%
Niacin	2 mg	13%
Iron	0.5 mg	3%
Zinc	0.4 mg	4%
Manganese	0.1 mg	4%
Sodium	130 mg	6%

*Percent Daily Values are base on a 2,000 calorie diet
† Daily Value not established

EACH SERVING CONTAINS
Proprietary Blend of Superfoods

VEGAN PROTEIN / SUPERFOODS BLEND	*18750* mg †

Pea Protein, Agave Inulin, Hemp Protein, Natural Vanilla Flavor, Guar Gum, Coconut Cream Milk Powder, Kale, Spinach, Beetroot, Luo Han Guo Berry Extract (Monk Fruit), DigeZyme®, Apple, Carrot, Pumpkin, Parsley, Tomato, Broccoli, Himalayan Pink Salt

Contains: Tree Nuts

8 97239 00204 8

Slim Blend Pro is a delicious and sugar-free 5-in-1 organic superfood powder that will support your immune system and help you meet your energy, fiber, protein, and micronutrient requirements. Try adding it to your daily juices to support nutrification and detoxification.

13. Stay Lean

Stay Lean

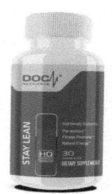

Stay Lean

- Suppress Appetite
- Support Improved Metabolism
- Support Healthy Weight Loss

Nitrogenous base and driving ingredients: *Irvingia Gabonensis Seed Extract, Guarana Seed Extract, Caralluma Fimbrata Aerial Parts Extract, Kudzu Root Powder, RNA, DNA.* **Other Ingredients:** *Hypromellose, (capsule), Rice Flour.*

14. Stem Cell Strong

Stem Cell Strong is a potent anti-aging powder that contains nearly 20 powerhouse herbs for optimizing health and restoring a sense of youthful virility. It contains Maca, Long Jack and Velvet Antler to boost testosterone and turbocharge libido; and l-citrulline to enhance blood flow to the` sex organs. It also contains a blend of powerful antioxidants to slow the aging process and adaptogenic herbs (ginkgo, ginseng, 5 potent mushrooms etc.) which will boost your energy and stamina both inside and outside of the bedroom. We are being asked by popular demand to bring this amazing supplement back on the market (expected by January 2021).

Supplement Facts

Serving Size 2 scoops (9.5g)
Servings Per Container 30

	Amount Per Serving	% Daily Value
Calories ††	30	
Total Fat	1 g	2%*
Total Carbohydrate	4 g	1%*
Dietary Fiber	1 g	6%*
Sugars	0 g	
Protein	2 g	
Vitamin A	731 IU	15%
Vitamin C	19 mg	32%
Vitamin K	5 mcg	6%
Niacin	1 mg	7%
Folate	9 mcg	2%
Vitamin B12	1 mcg	9%
Calcium	20 mg	2%
Iron	1 mg	6%
Phosphorus	77 mg	8%
Iodine	3 mcg	2%
Magnesium	34 mg	9%
Selenium	1 mcg	1%
Manganese	1 mg	55%
Sodium	0 mg	0%
Potassium	95 mg	3%
Proprietary Delgado Blend	5272 mg*	

(Rice Bran, Pumpkin Seed, Organic Cabbage, Cauliflower, Organic Maca, Glucosamine Sulfate, Nettle Leaf Powder, MSM, L-Citrulline Malate, LongJack , Ginger Root, Horny Goat Weed, Tart Cherry, American Ginseng, Ginkgo Biloba, Resveratrol)

Functional Sweet Blend (Carob, Stevia, Cacao)	2442 mg*
Sprouted Blend (Activated Barley Sprout and Oat Sprout)	1418 mg*
Algae Blend (Organic Spirulina, Blue Green Algae)	196 mg*
Proprietary Organic Mushroom Blend (Cordyceps, Reishi, Maitake, Lion's Mane, Tremella)	172 mg*

Other:
Magnesium Ascorbate, Manganese Gluconate

*Percent Daily Values are based on a 2000 calories diet
†Daily value not established

†† *These statements have not been evaluated by the Food and Drug Administration. This product is not intended to diagnose, treat, cure, or prevent any disease.*

In the event of a serious adverse event please contact us.

15. Testro Genin Cream

This is our most potent clinical strength cream and it uses a natural base for delivery of androgen-enhancing herbs. It is excellent for women who weigh over 180 lb, and according to a large-scale, five-year long pilot study, an ingredient in Testro Genin cream may successfully target cellulite. It's also beneficial for men accustomed to being more like an "alpha male."

Testro Genin™

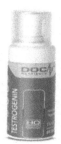

Benefits of Testro GeninTM:

- Can be used as part of a male sexual support protocol, a sports performance protocol, a Premenstrual Syndrome protocol, and an osteoporosis protocol.
- Naturally supports testosterone, healthy libido, and healthy bone density in men and women.

Proprietary blend (640mg): Astragalus *(Astragalus membranaceus)* Root, Oat Straw (*Avena Sativa*) Herb Extract 4:1, Catuaba Bark, Rhodiola Crenulata Root, Cordyceps Sinensis, Long Jack (*Eurycoma Longifolia*) Fruit Extract 200:1, Nettle Leaf , Tribulus Terrestris Fruit, Asian Ginseng (*Panax Ginseng*) Root, Muira Puama (*Ptychopetalum olacoide*) Bark, MACA Root, Velvet Bean (*Mucuna Prureins*) Seed, Horny Goat Weed (*Epimedium Sagittatum*) Extract 20% Icariin, Sea Buckthorn (*Hippophae rhamnoides*)Berry, Sea Cucumber, Cinnamon Bark, Red Sage(*Salvia Miltiorrhiza*) Root, Artichoke (*Cynara Scolymus*) Leaf, Rice Flour. Vegetable Capsules. **Active Ingredients**: RDA, Zinc Aspartate 5 mg (from Zinc sulfate 3 mg, Zinc gluconate 2 mg), Boron 0.5mg.

16. TestroGenesis

TestroGenesis cream contains 5-A-Hydroxy-Laxogenin which increases the natural production of your free and total testosterone. It also contains bioavailable zinc, DIM, pregnenolone, and DHEA to clear out toxic estrogens and bolster your immune system, as well as the natural antivirals -- alpha-lipoic acid, lavender, and vitamin B2. Because it is a cream, it gets directly absorbed through your skin into your bloodstream, which leads to immediate and notable results.

This cream is particularly beneficial for adults over the age of 50 who have naturally declined testosterone levels and should be applied daily to the neck and chest.

17. Testro Plus

This formula contains several herbs that boost testosterone and activate your body's natural defense system, as well as three different types of bioavailable zinc to further boost your immune system.

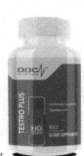

Testro Plus

Benefits of Pure Testro Plus ™:

- Can be used as part of a male sexual support protocol, a sports performance protocol, a Premenstrual Syndrome protocol, and an osteoporosis protocol.
- Naturally supports testosterone, healthy libido, and healthy bone density in men and women.

Proprietary Blend: *Astragalus Root, Oat Straw Herb Extract, Catuaba Bark, Rhodiola Crenulata Root Powder, Cordyceps Whole Mushroom Powder, Eurycoma Longifolia (Long Jack) Root Extract, Stinging Nettle Leaf Powder, Tribulus Fruit Powder, Asian Ginseng Root Powder, Muira Puama Bark Powder, Maca Root Powder, Velvet Bean Seed Powder, Epimedium Stem and Leaf Extract, Sea Buckthorn Berry Powder, Sea Cucumber Powder, Cassia Bark Powder, Chinese Salvia Root, Artichoke Leaf Powder.* **Other Ingredients**: *Hypromellose (capsule) Rice Flour.* **Active Ingredients**: *Zinc Aspartate 5 mg (from Zinc sulfate 3 mg, Zinc Gluconate 2 mg), Boron (as Boron Citrate) 0.5mg.*

18. Thyrodine

Thyrodine contains organic iodine and l-tyrosine - two essential nutrients for the thyroid that support those with under-functioning thyroids (hypothyroidism). Iodine is a mineral that has potent anti-viral properties and it helps the body to use oxygen. The World Health Organization states over 70% of adults are deficient in it.

Thyroidine™

About the Thyroid

Responsible for controlling our body's metabolism and organ function. The World Health Organization estimates about 1 billion people in the world are at high risk for thyroid problems. Often thyroid levels show "normal" and appropriate to the reference range, but Dr. Thierry Hertoghe, President of the International Hormone society warns most doctors don't test T3 which is completely imperative to our bodies. T3 once disregarded as unimportant because it is found in such small amounts, is now believed to be the most bioactive and important form of thyroid.

Low or high thyroid can cause:

- Low Energy / Fatigue
- Cold Hands and Feet
- Weight Gain
- Poor Mental Clarity
- Hair Loss
- Depression

Benefits of RAD Iodine:

- Thyroid Support
- Healthy Weight Support
- Healthy Metabolism Support
- Radiation Defense

2. 35 Questions to Build A Powerful Immune System

Foods to Avoid to Increase White Blood Cell Efficiency

Greasy high fat, refined carbohydrates, and excessive animal proteins slow the immune system because they are viewed as foreign proteins and thicken blood

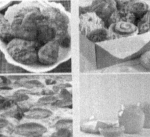

Fried Chicken

Filled with free radicals from the high heat cooking of processed flour, processed oil, and animal protein you basically can't get any worse unless you covered it in cheese

Baked Goods and Pastries

Processed sugar, processed oil, and processed flour make the unholy trinity of chronic disease

Pizza

Loads of cheese, deli meats, processed oil and refined carbohydrates stripped of fiber and nutritional value make pizza a dangerous dinner guest

Ghee(Clarified Butter)

Thought of as healthy by many especially of the keto crowd. But on a mechanical level it gums up the lymphatics immediately lowering white blood cell effectiveness

---

Claude Bernard was a 19th-century French physician and physiologist who stated: "The pathogen is nothing, the terrain is everything." This is pertinent because viruses in healthy bodies do not produce symptoms or cause damage. Only viruses that reproduce in an unhealthy terrain with toxic cells are pathogenic.[127] Even the famous Virologist Dr Sabin on his deathbed admitted the terrain is everything, saying "I was wrong, the microbe is not the danger, it is the care of the body to support a strong immune system."

---

[127] https://www.virology.ws/2004/07/28/what-is-a-virus/

If we support the immune system and modify our lifestyles to optimize "the terrain," a virus has less of a chance. Below are 35 questions to assess your level of protection. Questions you answer "no" to are weak spots in your health and immunity and things you need to start doing.

35 Questions to Determine Your Risk:

1. Do you abstain in most cases from eating animal products - including meat, poultry, fish, dairy, and eggs? (limit to less than no more than once a week or at best once a month)
2. Do you eat a whole-food, plant-based oil-free diet rich in omega fatty acids?
3. Do you consume at least 15 servings of vegetables and fruits daily?
4. Do you drink at least 9 cups of filtered water a day if you're a woman, or 12 if you are a man?[128] The amount of added water will vary depending on whether you consume a significant amount of blended or cold vegetable press juices, mostly plant-based diet, your health status, level of physical activity and the climate you live in -- but your

---

[128] https://www.mayoclinic.org/healthy-lifestyle/nutrition-and-healthy-eating/in-depth/water/art-20044256

urine should be clear. If it is yellow (and you aren't taking B vitamins that add a yellow hue to urine within minutes of consumption) you need to hydrate more.

5. Do you exercise for at least 30 minutes to 90 minutes a day?

6. Is your exercise regime balanced and does it include cardio, strength training, rebounding, and stretching?

7. Do you get at least 15 minutes of skin exposure to sunlight daily? If not, are you taking a 5,000 IU D3 vitamin supplement daily? The typical supplement with D2 is not recommended because it is synthetic and not as bioavailable. See Appendix.

8. Is your pH level at least 7.4, as determined by pH testing strips used on the first urination of the day?

9. Do you drink fresh green juice daily? The consumption of 64 ounces a day of beetroot and green vegetable drinks will optimize your immune defenses.

10. Do you consume large amounts of cruciferous vegetables in order to optimize your hormonal balance and prevent estrogen dominance? If not, do you take a DIM containing supplement?

11. Do you support brain, skin, immune system and cell membrane health with essential fatty

acids from whole foods that *aren't* stripped of their fiber, e.g. soaked nuts and seeds, olives, avocados, and coconut?

12. Do you avoid all oils, including olive oil, coconut oil, corn oil, and butter? It is ok to apply oil to your skin as the absorption of .01%, according to Press shown to relieve any fatty acid deficiency, will not clog up your blood flow.

13. Are you gargling with sea salt water upon waking and before going to bed?

14. Are you breaking a sweat for at least 10 minutes daily, either through exercise or infrared saunas?

15. Do you limit your consumption of alcohol to no more than one serving daily?

16. Do you abstain from tobacco products?

17. Do you avoid caffeinated beverages including coffee, tea, and energy drinks (if you need to boost your energy, stamina and brainpower take Adrenal DMG).

18. Do you avoid all sugar-containing and artificially sweetened beverages?

19. Do you avoid over the counter drugs such as NSAIDs, cough suppressants, sleeping pills, and heartburn products?

20. Do you release your bowels at least four to six times a day?

21. Do you consume at least 60 to 120 grams of fiber daily to clear out toxins and excess hormones and support healthy gut bacteria?

22. Do you support your antioxidant bodily needs daily with daily tablets of molecular hydrogen, H2, or an Echo water Hydrogen device?

23. Do you practice stress reduction techniques daily e.g. gentle yoga, meditation, breathwork, tai chi and neuro reprogramming?

24. Do you tell your family and friends or show them with acts of service how much you love them on a regular basis?

25. Are you and your partner intimate at least 5 times a week? Do you at least hug your pet?

26. Is your sex life mutually blissful and orgasmic? If not take my Mastering Love, Sex, and Intimacy course, it retails at $350, but is currently being offered for **$19**.

27. Do you use an Air Fresh ionizer (Everest is highly recommended) to clear pollutants out of your home?

28. Do you support stem cell production and mitochondrial functioning daily with a nutraceutical that contains medicinal mushrooms, velvet antler, and stem cell boosting herbs? For a clinically effective nutraceutical get Stem Cell Enhancer.

29. Do you protect yourself from EMF radiation by keeping phones out of the bedroom, using an EMF shield, and connecting with the earth at least twice a week (e.g. walking on the beach or in a forest)? We suggest the use of DNA Protector.

30. Do you fortify and alkalize your blood and body with a blend of superfood antioxidants, probiotics, essential fatty acids, and digestive enzymes? (Try Slim Blend Pro).

31. Do you detoxify regularly with Epsom salt or clay baths?

32. Do you practice gratitude throughout the day, focusing on all the blessings in your life and actively steering away from negative thinking?

33. Do you get at least eight hours of sleep at night, waking without an alarm and or taking an afternoon siesta or 30-minute to one-hour mediation break?

34. Do you use sleep hygiene measures to ensure your sleep is of high-quality, e.g. keeping electronics out of the bedroom, sleeping in a cool, dark, and silent environment, going to bed, and waking at the same time, etc.

35. Is your mind working *for* you? If you are experiencing stress, anxiety, fear, depression, or other negative emotions, your mind is working *against* you. These emotions

compromise the immune system and they need to be dealt with. Instead of focusing on the negative, make the decision to empower yourself with information so you can uplevel your health and vitality. Look into NickDelgado.com high level coaching with TimeLine Therapy to release negative values and limiting decisions.

5 Ways To Build Your Immune System: SHINE

1. Sleep & Stress Management
2. Hormones and Peptides
3. Infection Immunity
4. Nutrition and Nutraceutical Support
5. Exercise

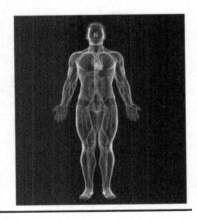

3. Life with a Purpose

Who are you? Why are you here? Why does it matter that you were born? The thoughts that pop into your head, your imaginings when your mind is drifting, are the preview of what's about to happen!

These thoughts come from your subconscious mind, that invisible part of you, the most important part, the power to do more than you can ever imagine. You <u>have</u> the power to achieve greatness. Go deep within and allow that small inner voice to tell you who you really are! You were born for a purpose, to stand out -- yes, you!

There is a part of you that most will never know. Your past can no longer hold you in bondage if you let go of limiting faulty beliefs about yourself and replace them with love, personal development, and contribution.

What dream have you forgotten? Give yourself permission to live your dream. As you allow your dreams to free your mind, live your beliefs, and change the way you act, there will be moments when you might say, "I can't believe I am really doing this!" What would you do if failure were not an option? What if your age or money were not a limit? Your dream has no possibility of failure, it has no artificial limits, such as age or finances. By thinking as you want to be, you will become your dream.

All dreams are accomplished first in the mind because the imagination is a preview of what will come. There is work for you, assigned only to you, and if you don't do it this dream will not become reality. This is your mission, your time.

To do something no one has done, you must release the fear that has held you back. The radical change you must make is to develop the courage to be a force of the truth, to see what that truth is. See yourself smiling and know that victory is yours.

You will have challenges to bring out the best in you, so always <u>be</u> at your best. The passion is in you to control your destiny! No force or obstacle will stop you if you believe that we attract the people who will bring you answers and people who will open doors you did not see.

The thoughts we focus on direct who we become, so let go of negative thoughts and reframe those thoughts to empower you and others. Lean into "bigger than life" projects as they come. Remember that there is only the moment that now exists. Live to be great and the answer will come.

Believe in your happiest dreams as you meditate and calm yourself and align yourself with your values and goals. Affirm to yourself each day, "I have dreams, talents, and resources that the world needs. I am the vessel to lead the world so that they can become the hero of their own lives."

It's your time, it's your hour -- you are chosen to succeed and live your dreams with rewards of life. Hereafter the level of distracting thoughts must be discarded to bring a journey of anticipation with the real you the higher self.

Greatness is a choice you must make every day. It will not come from the media nor your history. You will now learn to live out of your incredible imagination where you reside. And the key is meditating and dreaming big: the words, actions, and thoughts of that powerful spirit, your soul, within you.

Achieve things you have not even thought of yet as you listen to the moments between your thoughts - what <u>will</u> matter because you were born? What <u>will</u> cause you to stand out, to be chosen?

Consistency is the key to success. Be fearless every day, let go of your fear of failure or fear of success - or even "fear of missing out." Prepare yourself to be in a great relationship, a rewarding career with purpose, and be physically and emotionally strong, with forgiveness, humility, and compassion.

Where will you be in five years, ten years, or even twenty years from now by living your life in a big way? Healthy body, healthy mindset! You now have permission to live your dream by becoming and accepting that person you know you can be.

There is a change we are to make today and every day, and we must have the courage to see it, feel it, and do it with exhilaration and celebrate it with our loved ones. Yes, all dreams are accomplished with imagination.

Dr. Nick